Health
and the American Indian

Health and the American Indian has been co-published simultaneously as *Journal of Health & Social Policy,* Volume 10, Number 4 1999.

The *Journal of Health & Social Policy* Monographic "Separates"

Below is a list of "separates," which in serials librarianship means a special issue simultaneously published as a special journal issue or double-issue *and* as a "separate" hardbound monograph. (This is a format which we also call a "DocuSerial.")

"Separates" are published because specialized libraries or professionals may wish to purchase a specific thematic issue by itself in a format which can be separately cataloged and shelved, as opposed to purchasing the journal on an on-going basis. Faculty members may also more easily consider a "separate" for classroom adoption.

"Separates" are carefully classified separately with the major book jobbers so that the journal tie-in can be noted on new book order slips to avoid duplicate purchasing.

You may wish to visit Haworth's website at . . .

http://www.haworthpressinc.com

. . . to search our online catalog for complete tables of contents of these separates and related publications.

You may also call 1-800-HAWORTH (outside US/Canada: 607-722-5857), or Fax: 1-800-895-0582 (outside US/Canada: 607-771-0012), or e-mail at:

getinfo@haworthpressinc.com

Health and the American Indian, edited by Priscilla A. Day, MSW, and Hilary N. Weaver, DSW (Vol. 10, No. 4, 1999). *Discusses the health and mental health of Native American Indians from several aspects.*

Reason and Rationality in Health and Human Services Delivery, edited by John T. Pardeck, PhD, ACSW, Charles F. Longino, Jr., PhD, and John W. Murphy, PhD (Vol. 9, No. 4, 1998). *"A variety of perspectives that successfully challenge the pillars of modern medicine . . . . This book should be required of all health care professionals, especially those training to become physicians."* (Roland Meinert, PhD, President, Missouri Association for Social Welfare, Jefferson City, Missouri)

Selected Practical Problems in Health and Social Research, edited by Thomas E. Dinero, PhD (Vol. 8, No. 1, 1996). *"Explores some of the theoretical ideas underlying classical and modern measurement theory. These ideas form a set of guidelines for researchers, health professionals, and students in the social, psychological, or health sciences who are planning and evaluating a measurement activity."* (Inquiry)

Psychosocial Aspects of Sickle Cell Disease: Past, Present, and Future Directions of Research, edited by Kermit B. Nash, PhD (Vol. 5, No. 3/4, 1994). *"An excellent contribution to a neglected area of study and practice. . . . Offer[s] tools and techniques that one can easily incorporate into practice. Novice readers as well as seasoned practitioners will find the practicality of the book extremely helpful."* (Social Work in Health Care)

Health Care for the Poor and Uninsured: Strategies That Work, edited by Nellie P. Tate, PhD, and Kevin T. Kavanagh, MD, MS (Vol. 3, No. 4, 1992). *"Chapters are short and to the point with clearly defined goals, methods, techniques, and impacts and include easy-to-comprehend charts and statistics. This book will prove useful in understanding activities that may soon be an integral part of the American health care system."* (Journal of Community Health)

Health and the American Indian

Priscilla A. Day, MSW
Hilary N. Weaver, DSW
Editors

Health and the American Indian has been co-published simultaneously as *Journal of Health & Social Policy,* Volume 10, Number 4 1999.

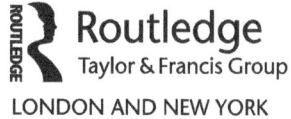

LONDON AND NEW YORK

First published 1999 by The Haworth Press, Inc.

2 Park Square, Milton Park, Abingdon, Oxon OX14 4RN
711 Third Avenue, New York, NY 10017, USA

Routledge is an imprint of the Taylor & Francis Group, an informa business

First issued in paperback 2016

Copyright © 1999 Taylor & Francis

Transferred to Digital Printing 2009 by Routledge

Health and the American Indian has been co-published simultaneously as *Journal of Health & Social Policy*™, Volume 10, Number 4 1999.

All rights reserved. No part of this book may be reprinted or reproduced or utilised in any form or by any electronic, mechanical, or other means, now known or hereafter invented, including photocopying and recording, or in any information storage or retrieval system, without permission in writing from the publishers.

Notice:
Product or corporate names may be trademarks or registered trademarks, and are used only for identification and explanation without intent to infringe.

Cover design by Thomas J. Mayshock Jr.

Library of Congress Cataloging-in-Publication Data

Health and the American Indian / Priscilla A. Day, Hilary N. Weaver, editors.
    p. cm.
    "Co-published simultaneously as Journal of health & social policy, volume 10, number 4, 1999."
    Includes bibliographical references and index.
    ISBN 0-7890-0658-8 (alk. paper)
    1. Indians of North America–Health and hygiene. 2. Indians of North America–Medical care. 3. Health–Cross-cultural studies. 4. Health and race–United States. I. Day, Priscilla A. II. Weaver, Hilary N. III. Journal of health & social policy.

RA448.5.I5H416 1999
362.1'089'97073–dc21
                                                                        99-12963
                                                                           CIP

Publisher's Note
The publisher has gone to great lengths to ensure the quality of this reprint but points out that some imperfections in the original may be apparent.

ISBN 978-0-7890-0658-5 (hbk)
ISBN 978-1-138-97584-2 (pbk)

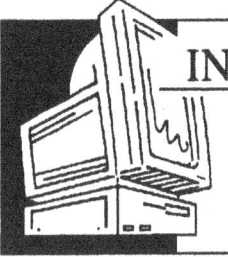

INDEXING & ABSTRACTING

Contributions to this publication are selectively indexed or abstracted in print, electronic, online, or CD-ROM version(s) of the reference tools and information services listed below. This list is current as of the copyright date of this publication. See the end of this section for additional notes.

- *Abstracts in Anthropology*

- *Academic Abstracts/CD-ROM*

- *BIOBUSINESS: covers business literature related to the life sciences; covers both business & life science periodicals in such areas as pharmacology, health care, biotechnology, foods & beverages, etc.*

- *BUBL Information Service, an Internet-based Information Service for the UK higher education community*

- *Cambridge Scientific Abstracts*

- *CNPIEC Reference Guide: Chinese National Directory of Foreign Periodicals*

- *EMBASE/Excerpta Medica Secondary Publishing Division*

- *Family Studies Database (online and CD/ROM)*

- *GEO Abstracts (GEO Abstracts/GEOBASE)*

- *Health Care Literature Information Network/HECLINET*

- *Health Management Information Service (HELMIS)*

- *Health Source: Indexing & Abstracting of 160 selected health related journals, updated monthly*

- *Health Source Plus: expanded version of "Health Source" to be released shortly*

- *Healthcare Marketing Abstracts*

- *HealthPromis*

(continued)

- *HealthSTAR*
- *Hospital and Health Administration Index*
- *IBZ International Bibliography of Periodical Literature*
- *Index to Periodical Articles Related to Law*
- *International Political Science Abstracts/Documentation Politique Internationale*
- *Medical Benefits*
- *Mental Health Abstracts (online through DIALOG)*
- *National Clearinghouse for Primary Care Information (NCPCI)*
- *NIAAA Alcohol and Alcohol Problems Science Database (ETOH)*
- *OT BibSys*
- *PAIS (Public Affairs Information Service) NYC*
- *Sage Public Administration Abstracts (SPAA)*
- *Social Planning/Policy & Development Abstracts (SOPODA)*
- *Social Work Abstracts*
- *Sociological Abstracts (SA)*
- *UP-TO-DATE Publications*
- *World Agricultural Economics & Rural Sociology Abstracts*

(continued)

*Special Bibliographic Notes related to special journal issues
(separates) and indexing/abstracting:*

- indexing/abstracting services in this list will also cover material in any "separate" that is co-published simultaneously with Haworth's special thematic journal issue or DocuSerial. Indexing/abstracting usually covers material at the article/chapter level.

- monographic co-editions are intended for either non-subscribers or libraries which intend to purchase a second copy for their circulating collections.

- monographic co-editions are reported to all jobbers/wholesalers/approval plans. The source journal is listed as the "series" to assist the prevention of duplicate purchasing in the same manner utilized for books-in-series.

- to facilitate user/access services all indexing/abstracting services are encouraged to utilize the co-indexing entry note indicated at the bottom of the first page of each article/chapter/contribution.

- this is intended to assist a library user of any reference tool (whether print, electronic, online, or CD-ROM) to locate the monographic version if the library has purchased this version but not a subscription to the source journal.

- individual articles/chapters in any Haworth publication are also available through the Haworth Document Delivery Service (HDDS).

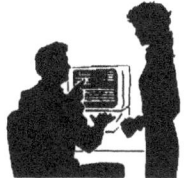

Health and the American Indian

CONTENTS

Gender Differences in the Historical Trauma Response
   Among the Lakota   1
    Maria Yellow Horse Brave Heart, PhD

At What Cost? The Social Impact
   of American Indian Gaming   23
    Thomas D. Peacock, EdD
    Priscilla A. Day, MSW
    Robert B. Peacock, MEd

Protecting the Future of Indigenous Children and Nations:
   An Examination of the Indian Child Welfare Act   35
    Hilary N. Weaver, DSW
    Barry J. White, MA

Whose Genes Are They? The Human Genome
   Diversity Project   51
    Leota Lone Dog, BA

Interactions Between American Indian Ethnicity
   and Health Care   67
    Wynne DuBray, PhD
    Adelle Sanders, MSW

Index   85

ABOUT THE EDITORS

Priscilla A. Day, MSW, is Assistant Professor of Social Work and Director, American Indian Projects at the University of Minnesota, Duluth. A member of the Leech Lake Reservation in Northern Minnesota, Ms. Day continues to work with American Indians on reservations as well as in urban areas. She is a member of the Council of Social Work Education, the National Indian Education Association, and a Bush Foundation Leadership Fellow. In addition, Ms. Day is a doctoral candidate in Educational Administration at the University.

Hilary N. Weaver, DSW, is Assistant Professor in the School of Social Work at the State University of New York at Buffalo. Her academic interests focus around social work with Native American Indians. Dr. Weaver is President of the American Indian Social Work Educators' Association and frequently gives presentations and workshops on indigenous issues and incorporating cultural factors into the helping process. In addition, she is Chair of the Native American Caucus of the National Association of Social Workers. Presently, Dr. Weaver is continuing research on comparative indigenous issues, which she started as a Visiting Scholar at the University of Waikato in New Zealand.

Gender Differences in the Historical Trauma Response Among the Lakota

Maria Yellow Horse Brave Heart, PhD

SUMMARY. The historical trauma response is a constellation of characteristics associated with massive cumulative group trauma across generations, similar to those found among Jewish Holocaust survivors and descendants. Trauma response features include elevated mortality rates and health problems emanating from heart disease, hypertension, alcohol abuse, and suicidal behavior. This article explores gender differences in the historical trauma response among the Lakota (Teton Sioux) and the correlation with health and mental health statistics.

The theory of a Lakota historical trauma response is first explained. Traditional gender roles are described in combination with modifications engendered by traumatic Lakota history. Then, data from a study on Lakota historical trauma are presented, including gender differences in response to an experimental intervention aimed at facilitating a trauma resolution process.

The data revealed significant gender differences. The sample of women presented initially with a greater degree of conscious affective experience of historical trauma. In contrast, the men reported more lifespan trauma associated with boarding school attendance and appeared to be at an earlier stage of grief. However, at the end of the intervention, women's experience of survivor guilt–a significant trauma response feature–decreased while men's consciousness of historical trauma and unresolved grief increased. Degree of traditional presentation-of-self, including phenotype, appeared to interact with gender to place male participants at greater risk for being traumatized over the lifespan and perhaps subsequently utilizing more rigid defenses against the con-

---

[Haworth co-indexing entry note]: "Gender Differences in the Historical Trauma Response Among the Lakota." Brave Heart, Maria Yellow Horse. Co-published simultaneously in *Journal of Health & Social Policy* (The Haworth Press, Inc.) Vol. 10, No. 4, 1999, pp. 1-21; and: *Health and the American Indian* (ed: Priscilla A. Day and Hilary N. Weaver) The Haworth Press, Inc., 1999, pp. 1-21. Single or multiple copies of this article are available for a fee from The Haworth Document Delivery Service [1-800-342-9678, 9:00 a.m. - 5:00 p.m. (EST). E-mail address: getinfo@haworthpressinc.com].

© 1999 by The Haworth Press, Inc. All rights reserved.

scious experience of the trauma with the exception of survivor guilt. The article concludes with a discussion of health and mental health implications for prevention and treatment of the trauma response which could positively impact the health status of the Lakota. Recommendations for future research are suggested. *[Article copies available for a fee from The Haworth Document Delivery Service: 1-800-342-9678. E-mail address: getinfo@haworthpressinc.com]*

The Lakota (Teton Sioux) *historical trauma response* is a constellation of characteristics associated with massive cumulative group trauma across generations, at least since the 1890 Wounded Knee Massacre, and is similar to traits identified for Jewish Holocaust descendants (Fogelman, 1988; Kestenberg, 1982/1990). Trauma response features include elevated mortality rates and health problems emanating from heart disease, hypertension, alcohol abuse, depression, and suicidal behavior. This article explores gender differences in the historical trauma response among the Lakota and the correlation with health and mental health statistics.

The article begins with a description of historical trauma theory in which traditional gender roles as well as the modifications engendered by traumatic Lakota history are briefly examined. Literature on health and mental health problems and their association with trauma are explored, including available data on gender differences, and other risk factors associated with trauma for American Indians are examined. Then, gender is explored in data from a small quantitative study on Lakota historical trauma including an examination of an intervening variable, degree of traditional presentation-of-self. The article concludes with a discussion of prevention, early identification, and intervention of the trauma response which could positively impact the health status of the Lakota. Recommendations for future research are suggested.

THE LAKOTA HISTORICAL TRAUMA RESPONSE

Lakota historical trauma is defined as cumulative and collective emotional and psychological injury both over the life span and across generations, resulting from a cataclysmic history of genocide. It is analogous to other massive generational group trauma features and is grounded in the trauma literature (van der Kolk, 1987, 1996). The constellation of features that appear in reaction to this traumatic history is called the Lakota historical trauma response (Brave Heart, 1998). The attending *historical unresolved grief* that results from the cumulative trauma is the impaired or delayed mourning that is part of the experience of massive loss.

Need for a Lakota Historical Trauma Response Theory

Standard Post-traumatic Stress Disorder (PTSD) nomenclature (American Psychiatric Association, 1994) fails to adequately represent American Indian trauma (Robin, Chester, & Goldman, 1996). Despite the extent of trauma reported in several studies of American Indian youth with close to two thirds affirming the experience of trauma and the respondents' perception of being seriously impacted by that trauma, many American Indian youth do not meet all of the diagnostic criteria for PTSD (Jones, Dauphinais, Sack, & Somervell, 1997; Manson, Beals, O'Nell, Piasecki, Bechtold, Keane, & Jones, 1996). Manson et al. (1996) raise questions about (a) cultural bias in the PTSD criteria and assessment instruments, (b) the possibility of a higher threshold for clinical response due to the pervasiveness and frequency of trauma among American Indians, and (c) culture influencing symptom presentation or the determination of what is pathological. Robin et al. (1996) identify the need for a way to examine the impact of a single trauma within the context of multigenerational and community trauma. The concepts of a historical trauma response and historical unresolved grief are intended to be inclusive of massive, genocidal trauma across generations upon which life span trauma is superimposed. Further, the concept of historical unresolved grief may shed light upon the prevalence of major depression among American Indians and is congruent with the concept of a traumatic depression (Davidson & Fairbank, 1993; Robin et al., 1996). Rather than utilizing proposed concepts such as complex PTSD (Herman, 1993), the Lakota historical trauma response incorporates traumatic group experiences such as the Wounded Knee Massacre and cultural constructs around indigenous grief.

Lakota Historical Trauma Response Features

Trauma response features may be manifested psychologically in symptoms such as depression, suicide, and substance abuse, as well as somatically through heart disease and hypertension. Characteristics of the Lakota historical trauma response are congruent with those identified in the Jewish Holocaust survivor syndrome (Niederland, 1988) and survivor's child complex (Kestenberg, 1990) and include: (a) anxiety, (b) intrusive trauma imagery, (c) depression, (d) survivor guilt, (e) elevated mortality rates from cardiovascular diseases as well as suicide and other forms of violent death (Eitinger & Strom, 1973; Keehn, 1980; Nefzger, 1970; Sigal & Weinfeld, 1989), (f) identification with ancestral pain and deceased ancestors, (g) psychic numbing and poor affect tolerance, and (h) unresolved grief. These features have been identified among the Lakota in early personality studies (Erikson, 1963; Macgregor, 1946/1975; Nurge, 1970) and more recent studies (Brave Heart-Jordan, 1995; Brave Heart, 1998, 1999, in press-d).

TRADITIONAL GENDER ROLES AND RELATIONSHIPS

Traditionally, Lakota women have been esteemed in contrast to the presentation in much of the ethnographic literature (Allen, 1986; Brave Heart-Jordan, & DeBruyn, 1995). Sex roles were complementary and neither women nor children were viewed as property. Domestic violence and child abuse were not tolerated. Men were the protectors of the society. The Sacred Pipe and Lakota spiritual mores were brought by *Pte Sa Win*, the White Buffalo Calf Woman (Black Elk & Brown, 1953/1971). According to Powers (1986), oral history reveals that *Pte Sa Win* asked men (a) to share in the women's sorrow as women experience grief more deeply and carry the grief for the Nation and (b) to help women with caring for the children. Legend reveals a complementary view of traditional indigenous gender roles and relationships.

In an examination of current health-risk behaviors among the Lakota, Han, Hagel, Welty, Ross, Leonardson, and Keckler (1994) found that healthier women were more traditional–defined as having a greater degree of Lakota life style, blood, and language fluency–than less traditional women. In contrast, more acculturated males were healthier than more traditional men. The study concluded that acculturation was more stressful for women. In a study of well-educated working urban Indian women, Napholz (1995) found less depression among women who showed both masculine and feminine traits. Traditionally Lakota women are valued for being industrious and having fortitude which may be seen, in the European American paradigm, as masculine traits.

COMORBIDITY OF THE TRAUMA RESPONSE WITH OTHER DISORDERS

Psychiatric Disorders

Cumulative trauma and PTSD may influence high rates of other psychiatric disorders among American Indians who have an elevated incidence of childhood sexual abuse; this abuse is a significant risk factor for the development of substance abuse, depression, and/or anxiety disorders (Robin et al., 1996). Excessive rates of trauma among American Indian adults as well as youth have been confirmed by more recent research (Manson et al., 1996) as well as a prevalence of depression and substance abuse which are correlated with PTSD (Robin et al., 1996).

Depression and suicide: Comorbidity and gender. Depression is the most common co-morbid condition with PTSD (Ursano, Grieger, & McCarroll, 1996). Survivors of massive trauma often develop an identification with the dead in their unresolved grief, sometimes manifested in suicidal behavior (Bergmann & Jucovy, 1982/1990; Lifton, 1968, 1988). A study among the Oglala Lakota (May, 1973) reflected that those who attempted suicide exhibited a high incidence of loss over the life span. Van Winkle and May (1993) found that completed suicides are more prevalent among young Indian males while more attempters are female (Zitzow & Desjarlait, 1994). Chronic and complicated depression appeared to be more prevalent among Northern Plains Indians (Shore, Manson, Bloom, Keepers, & Neligh, 1987) which includes the Lakota.

The suicide rate is 27.9 per 100,000 for the Aberdeen Area Indian Health Service (IHS), which includes primarily Lakota and Dakota reservations, more than twice the rate of 11.4 for the United States' general population (IHS, 1995a). The suicide attempt rate on an unspecified Lakota reservation was almost seven times that of the United States' average (Claymore, 1988). The elevated suicide rates among the Lakota are a manifestation of unresolved grief and pathological identification with the dead (Brave Heart-Jordan, 1995; Brave Heart, 1998). In addition to unresolved grief from traumatic loss, suicide attempts and self-mutilation had high correlations with sexual abuse especially early in life (Herman & van der Kolk, 1987; Bachman, 1992).

Alcohol and/or other drug abuse. Among American Indians, substance abuse is associated with suicide (Bachman, 1992; Claymore, 1988) and childhood trauma (Robin et al., 1996). The alcoholism death rate is 89.3 per 100,000 for Indians in the Aberdeen Area compared with 6.8 for the United States (IHS, 1995). Robin et al. (1996) noted that the alcohol-related mortality rates for Indian women are three to five times higher than for women in the general United States population. Major depression was more prevalent among alcohol free Indian women than abstinent Indian men (Robin et al., 1996). However, liver disease and accident mortality, which are typically alcohol-related, are higher for men than for women (IHS, 1995b). American Indian females in residential treatment for substance abuse manifested a greater degree of family dysfunction including emotional, physical, and sexual abuse (Gutierres, Russo, & Urbanski, 1994). The possibility of abuses experienced outside of the family, i.e., in boarding schools, was unclear.

Medical and Psychosomatic Conditions

Premenstrual related disorders have been observed among American Indian women with life span trauma, particularly abusive boarding school experiences (Brave Heart, in press-c). Physical health has been a historical problem among the Lakota since the inception of Lakota reservations in 1871 (Tanner, 1982). Indian Health Service (1995a) revealed high rates of coronary heart disease as well as hypertension and accidental deaths, particularly among the Lakota. Untreated major depression and anxiety disorders (which are elevated among Native people) have a negative effect upon health status, with major depression having the greatest impact while PTSD is next (Schonfeld, Verboncoeur, Fifer, Lipschutz, Lubeck, & Buesching, 1997). There is an association between PTSD and somatization (Pribor, Yutzy, Dean, & Wetzel, 1993; Saxe, Chinman, Berkowitz, Hall, Lieberg, Schwartz, & van der Kolk, 1994). Additionally, somatic features and depression are highly correlated on the Center for Epidemiologic Studies-Depression Scale administered to American

Indian boarding school adolescents (Dick, Beals, Keane, & Manson, 1994) which suggests an association between these two. Psychic numbing and poor affect tolerance, common with PTSD, often result in the expression of feelings somatically.

Heart and cerebrovascular diseases. Among the Lakota, the leading cause of death for both genders is heart disease (IHS, 1995b). There is a higher prevalence of heart disease among men. However, women with diabetes had higher rates of coronary heart disease (Howard, Lee, Cowan, Fabsitz, Howard, Oopik, Robbins, Savage, Yeh, & Welty, 1995). The Aberdeen Area age-adjusted mortality rate from heart disease is 237.5 per 100,000, the highest of all Indian groups and almost twice the rate of the general United States population. Lakota have higher rates of morbidity and mortality from myocardial infarctions than the general population (Hrabovsky, Welty, & Coulehan, 1989), particularly among 25-44 year olds who have higher death rates than the United States population (Welty & Coulehan, 1993). Studies within the general population reveal a co-occurrence of heart disease and psychiatric diagnoses, especially depression and anxiety, both elevated among American Indians, as well as PTSD. Psychological factors influence the development and the medical course as well as prognosis of heart disease (Hamner, 1994; Shapiro, 1996).

Cerebrovascular diseases are higher for Indian women (IHS, 1995b). The cerebrovascular mortality rate is 47.4 for the Aberdeen Area, again the highest of all Indian Health Service regions; this is almost double the United States rate of 26.8 (IHS, 1995a).

Tuberculosis. The Aberdeen Area tuberculosis death rate of 5.6 is more than five times the United States rate (IHS, 1995a). While tuberculosis itself has not been associated with PTSD, the elevated mortality rates for the Lakota place this population at risk for additional health related trauma. Further, there is a historical legacy of massive tuberculosis deaths associated with the inception of boarding schools and the reservation system (Brave Heart-Jordan, 1995; Tanner, 1982). Gender differences were not reported.

GENDER DIFFERENCES IN TRAUMA RESPONSE RISK FACTORS

Risk factors are defined here as those conditions which may predispose someone to experiencing trauma. These factors include lower life expectancy and lower socioeconomic status, racism and oppression, and a history of generational as well as life span trauma such as boarding school attendance. Gender may interact with these risk factors and influence the presentation of symptoms. Interestingly, for another historically oppressed group, African American men showed the highest level of stress in response to trauma (Allen, 1996; Norris, 1992). This is congruent with findings that (a) men with PTSD were more likely to be substance dependent than women with PTSD (Manson et al., 1996) and (b) men have elevated suicide mortality despite women's higher attempt rates and greater incidence of major depression.

Life Expectancy and Socioeconomic Status

Premature death rates for American Indians are higher than the general population and African Americans; 31% of deaths occurred before age 45 compared with 23% for African Americans and 9% for Caucasian Americans (IHS, 1995b). This places American Indians at higher risk for traumatic grief from early losses.

Almost 50% (49.6%) of Indians in the Aberdeen Area live below the poverty level (IHS, 1995a). Unemployment is higher among Lakota males at 26.5% in the Aberdeen Area than for females at 19.4% (IHS, 1995a). On some Lakota reservations, the unemployment rate has been as high as 80% (Bureau of Indian Affairs, 1990), a substantial risk factor particularly for Lakota men. Albers (1983) identified the negative impact of European colonization upon the political status of Indian women under federal domination, gender differences in employment, and the economic balance of power between genders among the Dakotas.

Degree of Traditional Presentation-of-Self

For the purposes of this study, the degree of *traditional presentation-of-self* is utilized to include phenotype (skin color and features) as well as level of traditional identification or orientation, including fluency in Lakota. Traditional presentation-of-self may place one at more risk for racism and discrimination. Racism and oppression have been identified as conditions, coupled with traumatic group history, which may exacerbate PTSD among American Indians (Holm, 1994;

Manson et al., 1996; Silver & Wilson, 1988) and increase the frequency and affliction of PTSD among African Americans who also have elevated rates of hypertension and heart disease (Allen, 1996). Hughes and Hertel (1990) found that darker skin color negatively impacted the socioeconomic status of African Americans, those with lighter skin having higher status; lighter skin color is still preferred within the African American community (Hall, 1992). Research is needed on the role of skin color psychosocially and biologically in hypertension among African Americans (Thomas, 1984). Montalvo (1987) emphasizes the need for more research on the impact of skin color among Latinos. Indian identity, an aspect of the presentation-of-self, was an issue for Viet Nam veterans, many with PTSD. Indian soldiers identified with the Vietnamese, more phenotypically similar than the European American soldiers who represented the historical enemy–the cavalry (Holm, 1994; Manson et al., 1996; Silver & Wilson, 1988). More research on American Indian identity is needed (Weaver, 1996), including the examination of phenotype as an important construct.

HISTORICAL TRAUMA INTERVENTION AND METHODOLOGY

The historical trauma intervention was delivered to a group of 45 Lakota men and women service providers and community leaders, focusing on the cumulative trauma response through a brief intensive psychoeducational group experience (Brave Heart-Jordan, 1995; Brave Heart, 1998). Goals included imparting a sense of mastery and control (van der Kolk, McFarlane, & van der Hart, 1996), in spite of our oppression and cumulative historical traumatization, within a safe haven–our sacred *Paha Sapa* (Black Hills). Participants were exposed to historical traumatic memories as well as opportunities for cognitive integration, necessary for effective treatment (Resick & Schnicke, 1992). Small and large group process provided opportunities for verbalization of traumatic experiences which has been found to decrease psychosomatic symptoms (Harber & Pennebaker, 1992) as well as reduce psychic numbing and increase affect tolerance. Traditional Lakota culture and ceremonies were integrated throughout the intervention which have a curative effect on PTSD (Silver & Wilson, 1988).

Responses to the intervention were examined. Self-report measures were taken at three intervals. Data collection instruments included a demographic and trauma history questionnaire prior to the intervention (T1), a Lakota Grief Experience Questionnaire (LGEQ), adapted from Barrett and Scott (1989), at T1 and at the end of the intervention (T2), and the semantic differential (Osgood, Suci, & Tannenbaum, 1957/1978) T1 and T2. The semantic differential contained concepts or stimuli followed by bipolar word pairs and a rating scale to measure meaning in three dimensions: evaluation, potency, and activity. An evaluation form at T2 and a six week follow-up measure (T3) were also collected.

The data were analyzed for each instrument using measures of central tendency, frequency, and descriptive statistics. The semantic differential was examined using paired t-tests and t-tests for independent samples.

FINDINGS

Gender Differences in Trauma History and Response

The mean age of the reservation-based study population was 43 years; 59.1% were female. There was a 97.8% completion rate. More men attended boarding school (82.4%) than women (65.4%). Although women were placed in boarding schools at a higher mean distance (139.06 miles) than men (103.64 miles), men visited home less often with 57.1% visiting three or more times per year compared with 64.7% of the women. Other gender differences are illuminated in Table 1 and include the quality of boarding school experiences with men reporting more harsh treatment overall including being hit more often (85.7%) and being sexually abused more often (28.6%) than women (17.7%).

On the Lakota Grief Experience Questionnaire (LGEQ) at T1, women (75.0%) felt more responsible to undo the pain of the historical past than men (66.6%), but men experienced more guilt at having survived trauma (56.3%) than women (44.0%). Women experienced greater pain upon remembering traumatic history (92.0%) than men (85.7%). However, women avoided discussing boarding school trauma (37.5%) less than men (56.3%), yet more men (55.6%) perceived

TABLE 1. Gender Differences on Boarding School Experiences

	% Male	% Female
Attended boarding school	82.4%	65.4%
Hit at boarding school	85.7%	35.3%
Punished for speaking Indian language	57.1%	20.0%
Experienced racism in boarding school	85.7%	58.8%
Sexually abused at boarding school	28.6%	17.7%

themselves as talking openly about sad feelings than women (46.2%). Half of the sample of both men and women (50%) had experienced a death within the past year and 100% within the past two years.

Lakota historical trauma was experienced with significantly more potency by men at T1 on the semantic differential ($P = .001$, $p. < 01$). In contrast, anger was significantly more potent for women at T1 ($P = .046$, $p. < 05$).

Health problems included hypertension for 50% of all respondents. A family history of heart disease was reported by 27.9% of respondents but only 2.3%, all men, admitted this for themselves. A history of alcohol abuse was affirmed by a larger number of men (94.4%) than women (73.1%).

Gender Differences in Traditional Presentation-of-Self

I observed more fullblood men than women in the sample and more men (47.1%) reported fluency in Lakota than women (28.0%); parental Lakota fluency for men was 94.1% compared with women at 76.9%, further suggesting a greater number of fullblood men in the sample. The majority of Indian men perceived themselves as looking mostly Indian (67%). When asked if they saw themselves as looking purely Indian, despite the higher number of fullblood men than women, their response was low (1.1%) compared with women (28.0%). When the two categories were combined, more Indian men (68.1%) than women (28.0%) in the sample perceived themselves as having an Indian phenotype. However, more women practiced traditional spirituality (see Table 2).

TABLE 2. Gender Differences in Traditional Presentation-of-Self

	% Male	% Female
Looking purely or mostly Indian	61.1%	28.0%
Speak Indian	47.1%	28.0%
Parents spoke Indian	94.1%	76.9%
Actively participate in pow wows	61.1%	46.2%
Listen to Indian music often/frequently	44.4%	53.8%
Eat Indian food frequently	16.7%	23.1%
Wear Indian clothing/jewelry frequently	38.9%	32.0%
Practice Indian spirituality frequently	27.8%	53.8%

Gender Differences at T2

At the end of the intervention, all respondents (100%) felt the intervention was helpful in their historical trauma and unresolved grief resolution, with 78.8% indicating high agreement. All trauma related affects reduced by a rate of 50-100% after the intervention for the group as a whole including sadness, grief, anger, hopelessness, shame, helplessness, and guilt; positive affects such as joy and pride increased by more than 50% (Brave Heart-Jordan, 1995; Brave Heart, 1998). However, gender differences were apparent on the T2 evaluation, which had a 75% valid response rate. At T2, women's anger reduced more than men's. Women were less sad, felt less overall guilt (as opposed to survivor guilt), and shame at T2 than the men who felt more sadness, guilt, and shame. Joy increased for women but showed less of an increase over time than men who felt less joy at T1 but greater joy at T2 (see Table 3).

Although the group score on the LGEQ decreased, the overall grief score reduction did not meet significance, due to the diversity in response by gender. The women decreased in their overall grief score from 2.99 to 2.64 while men's grief score increased from 2.88 to 2.94. However, there were seven items that reduced over time with significance. Of the significant items on the LGEQ, there were observable gender differences for feeling responsible to undo the pain of the people's past. At T2 women felt less responsible (57.2%) while men felt more responsible (77.0%). Men experienced more survivor guilt at

TABLE 3. Group Totals and Gender Differences for Affects Experienced Often Before and After Intervention

Group	Before	After		
Sadness	66.7%	18.2%		
Grief	54.5	27.3		
Pride	51.5	81.8		
Anger	69.7	18.2		
Hopelessness	45.5	0.0		
Shame	60.6	6.1		
Helplessness	54.5	0.0		
Joy	45.5	75.8		
Guilt*	60.6	6.1		
Gender	Female	Male	Female	Male
	Before		After	
Anger	70.6%	73.3%	11.8%	26.7%
Sadness	70.6	66.7	5.9	33.3
Guilt*	70.6	53.3	0.0	13.3
Shame	64.7	60.0	0.0	13.3
Joy	58.8	33.3	70.6	86.7

*general, not specifically survivor guilt

both T1 (56.3%) and T2 (84.7%) than women whose survivor guilt decreased over time from 44.0% (T1) to 28.5% (T2) while men's increased. Additionally, there were contrasting directional changes for pain upon remembering tribal history with women decreasing from 92.0% (T1) to 85.7% (T2) while men's pain increased from 85.7% (T1) to 100% (T2). Further, although there was no change for women in their avoidance of discussing boarding school trauma–37.5% at T1 and T2–men's avoidance increased from 56.3% (T1) to 84.7% (T2).

At T2, there was a significant gender difference on one of the three semantic differential scales. T-tests for independent samples revealed a statistically significant gender difference at T2 on the evaluation scale for the concept *Wasicu* (White Man); women had a more positive score (M = 3.78) than men (M = 4.59) despite their more negative evaluation of this concept at T1. This gender difference was significant (P = .037, p < .05). Gender difference was also significant on the concept My True Self which changed on the potency (P = .004, p < .01) and evaluation (P = .035, p < .05) scales in a positive direction.

At T3, the follow-up evaluation return rate was 62.2%. A majority (89.3%) found the intervention had been very helpful in the resolution of historical unresolved grief and the remainder found it at least somewhat helpful. Gender differences were not assessed at T3.

DISCUSSION

Men—more fullblood Lakota in appearance and language—experienced greater trauma in boarding schools including more physical and sexual abuse and experienced greater sadness, survivor guilt, and shame as well as joy at T2. Hair length may have influenced men's limited self-appraisal of looking purely Indian; some fullblood men with short hair rated themselves as looking mostly Indian. Other explanations related to the complexity of Indian identity have been suggested to explain inaccurate self-image (Weaver & Brave Heart, 1999). With a greater degree of phenotypical Indian congruence than the women, men may have been placed at greater risk for compounding traumatic effects of racism. Further, men's historical inability to enact their traditional roles as protectors during the Wounded Knee Massacre, for example, may have heightened initial (T1) defensive denial of shame and general guilt (as opposed to survivor guilt) and lessened conscious awareness of the Lakota historical trauma and its impact. At the end of the intervention, men reported an increase in survivor guilt and shame as well as joy, suggesting an increase in affect tolerance and a decrease in psychic numbing as well as greater consciousness of trauma response features. The intervention may have served to move men from denial and trauma fixation to a later stage of resolution and imparted more tolerance and awareness of their survivor guilt.

In contrast, women's higher grief scores and sense of responsibility and general guilt at the outset of the intervention suggests a greater degree of awareness and perhaps less fixated grief, in keeping with *Pte Sa Win's* observation that the women would carry the grief for the Lakota. The intervention permitted women to relinquish some of their guilt (reduced by almost 100%) as well as grief. Perhaps the men also heeded the request of *Pte Sa Win* to help the women carry the grief, facilitated by the intervention's spiritual focus and emphasis on traditional Lakota mores.

Interestingly, the men's avoidance of discussing boarding school trauma increased after the intervention. One possible explanation for this response among the men in this sample is the stigma and shame associated with their more prevalent sexual abuse victimization, particularly for Lakota *wicasa* (men) who come from a legacy of warriors. Their shame is compounded by their failure, through no fault of their own, to be the protectors of the *Oyate* (Lakota Nation) and the intervention may have heightened their awareness of their traditional role and their impotence as well as their own victimization at Wounded Knee. Further, Lakota male reaction to trauma may mirror that of African American men who manifested a higher degree of stress in their trauma response (Allen, 1996; Norris, 1992) and hence, more avoidance. In contrast, the women entered the intervention with a greater level of participation in traditional spirituality which probably facilitated greater coping skills (deVries, 1996; Silver & Wilson, 1988).

It is unclear how much gender interacted with phenotype to influence the life span trauma and the response. Research on trauma risk factors including American Indian phenotype and its correlation with life span as well as generational trauma may elucidate features of gender differences in the trauma response. The role of gender is an important consideration in designing effective interventions for both women and men. Comorbidity of the Lakota historical trauma response with psychiatric and somatic conditions, which was not examined in the current study, also needs further exploration.

CONCLUSION

The theory of a Lakota historical trauma response must include examination of the differential effects of gender and traditional presentation-of-self, particularly phenotype, as well as investigation of the relationship with serious health problems among the Lakota. Increased affect tolerance from mastery of trauma may reduce somatization, thereby limiting the risk associated with coronary heart disease and hypertension. Further, trauma mastery can serve as a protective factor against physiological illness as well as depression and other psychiatric disorders. The integration of traditional spirituality and culture enhance protective factors against the development or exacerbation of PTSD (deVries, 1996; Silver & Wilson, 1988), facilitating prevention and treatment.

One challenge for healing the Lakota historical trauma response is the subjugation and distortion of historical facts about our genocide and the lack of awareness and sensitivity in the general population. As validation of the trauma and giving testimony are germane to the healing process, the lack of acknowledgment of our trauma is a barrier to our liberation from the effects of our historical legacy and the trauma response. This prohibition of the open expression of our traumatic affect and the lack of sufficient validation may increase health risk factors and predispose us to coronary heart disease, hypertension, suicide, and alcohol-related deaths. Theories of oppression which can lead to our self-destruction (Brave Heart & DeBruyn, in press) call for community education about and acknowledgment of our genocide to facilitate a healing process.

The *Takini* (Survivor) Network, a collective of Lakota traditional spiritual leaders and service providers, formed in *Paha Sapa* in 1992 to address healing from our historical trauma. With encouragement from the Jewish Holocaust survivor community, the Takini Network is conducting research, community education, and community healing aimed at validating our historical trauma and providing forums for Native people to begin to confront our traumatic past. It is imperative that we continue and expand this work as our people are in danger of increased trauma and elevated mortality rates in a cycle of risk. We must limit risk factors and develop protective factors through research, prevention, and intervention with historical trauma, for the Lakota Nation and other indigenous nations, *hecel lena oyate kin nipi kte*–so that the people may live!

REFERENCES

Albers, P. (1983). Sioux women in transition: A study of their changing status in a domestic and capitalist sector of production. In P. Albers & B. Medicine (Eds.), *The hidden half: Studies of Plains Indian women* (pp. 267-277). Lanham, MD & London: University Press of America.

Allen, I.M. (1996). PTSD among African Americans. In Marsella, A.J., Friedman, M.J., Gerrity, E.T., & Scurfield, R.M. (Eds.), *Ethnocultural aspects of post-traumatic stress disorder: Issues, research, and clinical applications*. Washington, DC: American Psychological Association, 209-238.

American Psychiatric Association. (1994). *Diagnostic and statistical manual of mental disorders* (4th ed.). Washington, DC.
Bachman, R. (1992). *Death and violence on the reservation: Homicide, family violence, and suicide in American Indian populations.* New York: Auburn House.
Barrett, T.W. & Scott, T.B. (1989). Development of the grief experience questionnaire. *Suicide and Life Threatening Behavior, 19*(2), 201-215.
Bergmann, M.S. & Jucovy, M.E. (Eds.) (1990). *Generations of the Holocaust.* New York: Columbia University Press. (original work published 1982).
Black Elk & Brown, J.E. (1971). *The Sacred Pipe.* Baltimore: Penguin Books. (original work published 1953).
Brave Heart-Jordan, M.Y.H. (1995). The return to the sacred path: Healing from historical trauma and historical unresolved grief among the Lakota. Doctoral dissertation, Smith College School for Social Work, 1995.*
Brave Heart-Jordan, M. & DeBruyn, L. M. (1995). So she may walk in balance: Integrating the impact of historical trauma in the treatment of Native American Indian women. In J. Adleman & G. Enguidanos (Eds.). *Racism in the lives of women: Testimony, theory, and guides to anti-racist practice* (pp. 345-368). New York: The Haworth Press, Inc.
Brave Heart, M.Y.H. (1998). The return to the sacred path: Healing the historical trauma and historical unresolved grief response among the Lakota. *Smith College Studies. 68*(3), 287-305
Brave Heart, M.Y.H. (1999). *Oyate Ptayela*: Rebuilding the Lakota Nation through addressing historical trauma among Lakota parents. *Journal of Human Behavior in the Social Environment. 2*(1/2), 109-126
Brave Heart, M.Y.H. (in press-c). Premenstrual dysphoric disorder among American Indian women: A preliminary exploration. *Rural Community Mental Health.*
Brave Heart, M.Y.H. (in press-d). *Wakiksuyapi*: Carrying the historical trauma of the Lakota. *Tulane Studies in Social Welfare.*
Brave Heart, M.Y.H. & DeBruyn, L.M. (1998). The American Indian Holocaust: Healing historical unresolved grief. *American Indian and Alaska Native Mental Health Research 8*(2), 56-78.
Bureau of Indian Affairs Labor Force Report (1990). Aberdeen, SD: Bureau of Indian Affairs.
Claymore, B. (1988). A public health approach to suicide attempts on a Sioux reservation. *American Indian and Alaska Native Mental Health Research, 1*(3), 19-24.
Davidson, R.T. & Fairbank, J.A. (1993). The epidemiology of post-traumatic stress disorder. In Davidson, R.T. & Foa, E.B. (Eds.), *Post-traumatic stress disorder: DSM IV and beyond* (pp. 147-169). Washington, DC: American Psychiatric Press.
deVries, M.W. (1996). Trauma in cultural perspective. In van der Kolk, B.A., McFarlane, A.C., & Weisaeth, L. (Eds.), *Traumatic stress: The effects of overwhelming experience on mind, body, and society.* New York: Guilford Press, pp. 398-413.

---

*Brave Heart-Jordan, 1995. Copyright by author. Reprints available through the Takini Network, c/o the author, University of Denver School of Social Work, 2148 S. High Street, Denver, CO 80208.

Dick, R.W., Beals, J., Keane, E.M., & Manson, S.M. (1994). Factorial structure of the CES-D among American Indian adolescents. *Journal of Adolescence, 17*(1), 73-79.

Eitinger, L. & Strom, A. (1973). *Mortality and morbidity after excessive stress: A follow-up investigation of Norwegian concentration camp survivors.* New York: Humanities Press.

Erikson, E. H. (1963). *Childhood and Society* (Rev. ed.). New York: W.W. Norton.

Fogelman, E. (1988). Therapeutic alternatives for Holocaust survivors and the second generation. In R. L. Braham (Ed.). *The psychological perspectives of the Holocaust and of its aftermath* (pp. 79-108). New York: Columbia University Press.

Gutierres, S.E., Russo, N.F., & Urbanski, L. (1994). Sociocultural and psychological factors in American Indian drug use: Implications for treatment. *International Journal of Addictions, 29*(14), 1761-1786.

Hall, R.E. (1992). Bias among African Americans regarding skin color: Implications for social work practice. *Research on Social Work Practice, 2*(4), 479-486.

Hamner, M.B. (1994). Exacerbation of Post-traumatic Stress Disorder symptoms with medical illness. *General Hospital Psychiatry, 16*(2), 135-137.

Han, P.K., Hagel, J., Welty, T.K., Ross, R., Leonardson, G., & Keckler, A. (1994). Cultural factors associated with health-risk behavior among the Cheyenne River Sioux. *American Indian and Alaska Native Mental Health Research, 5*(3), 15-29.

Harber, K.D. & Pennebaker, J.W. (1992). Overcoming traumatic memories. In S.A. Christianson (Ed.), *The handbook of emotion and memory: Research and theory* (pp. 359-386). Hillsdale, NJ: Erlbaum.

Herman, J.L. (1993). Sequelae of prolonged and repeated trauma: Evidence for a complex post-traumatic syndrome (DESNOS). In Davidson, R.T. & Foa, E.B. (Eds.), *Post-traumatic stress disorder: DSM IV and beyond* (pp. 213-228). Washington, DC: American Psychiatric Press.

Herman, J.L. & van der Kolk, B.A. (1987). Traumatic origins of borderline personality disorder. In B.A. van der Kolk (Ed.), *Psychological trauma.* Washington, DC: American Psychiatric Press.

Holm, T. (1994). The national survey of Indian Vietnam Veterans. *American Indian and Alaska Native Mental Health Research, 6*(3), pp. 18-28.

Howard, B.V., Lee, E.T., Cowan, L.D., Fabsitz, R.R., Howard, W.J., Oopik, A.J., Robbins, D.C., Savage, P.J., Yeh, J.L., & Welty, T.K. (1995). Coronary heart disease prevalence and its relation to risk factors in American Indians: The Strong Heart study. *American Journal of Epidemiology, 142*(3), 254-268.

Hrabovsky, S.L., Welty, T.K., & Coulehan, J.L. (1989). Acute myocardial infarction and sudden death in Sioux Indians. *Western Journal of Medicine, 150*(4), 420-422.

Hughes, M. & Hertel, B.R. (1990). The significance of color remains: A study of life chances, mate selection, and ethnic consciousness among Black Americans. *Social Forces, 68*(4), 1105-1120.

Indian Health Service (1995a). *Regional differences in Indian health.* Washington, DC: U.S. Department of Health and Human Services.

Indian Health Service (1995b). *Trends in Indian health.* Washington, DC: U.S. Department of Health and Human Services.

Jones, M.C., Dauphinais, P., Sacl, W.H., & Somervell, P.D. (1997). Trauma-related symptomatology among American Indian adolescents. *Journal of Traumatic Stress, 10*(2), 163-167.

Keehn, R.J. (1980). Follow-up studies of World War II and Korean conflict prisoners: Mortality to January 1, 1976. *American Journal of Epidemiology, III,* 194-202.

Kestenberg, J.S. (1990). A metapsychological assessment based on an analysis of a survivor's child. In M.S. Bergmann & M.E. Jucovy (Eds.), *Generations of the Holocaust* (pp. 137-158). New York: Columbia University Press. (original work published 1982).

Lifton, R.J. (1988). Understanding the traumatized self: Imagery, symbolization, and transformation. In J.P. Wilson, Z. Harel, & B. Kahana (Eds.), *Human adaptation to extreme stress: From the Holocaust to Vietnam* (pp. 7-31). New York: Plenum Press.

Lifton, R.J. (1968). *Death in life: Survivors of Hiroshima.* New York: Random House.

Macgregor, G.U. (1975). *Warriors without weapons: A study of the society and personality development of the Pine Ridge Sioux.* Chicago: University of Chicago Press (original work published 1946).

Manson, S., Beals, J., O'Nell, T., Piasecki, J., Bechtold, D., Keane, E., & Jones, M. (1996). Wounded spirits, ailing hearts: PTSD and related disorders among American Indians. In Marsella, A.J., Friedman, M.J., Gerrity, E.T., & Scurfield, R.M. (Eds), *Ethnocultural aspects of Post-traumatic Stress Disorder.* Washington, DC: American Psychological Association, pp. 255-283.

May, P. (1973). *Suicide and suicide attempts on the Pine Ridge Reservation.* Pine Ridge, SD: PHS Community Mental Health Program.

May, P. (1987). Suicide and self-destruction among American Indian youth. *American Indian and Alaska Native Mental Health Research, 1*(1), 52-69.

Montalvo, F.F. (1987). *Skin color and Latinos: The origins and contemporary patterns of ethnoracial ambiguity among Mexican Americans and Puerto Ricans.* San Antonio, TX: Institute for Intercultural Studies and Worden School of Social Work, Our Lady of the Lake University.

Napholz, L. (1995). Mental health and American Indian Women's Multiple Roles. *American Indian and Alaska Native Mental Health Research, 6*(2), 57-75.

Nefzger, M.D. (1970). Follow-up studies of World War II and Korean War prisoners: Study plan and mortality findings. *American Journal of Epidemiology, 91*(2), 123-138.

Niederland, W.G. (1988). The clinical aftereffects of the Holocaust in survivors and their offspring. In R.L. Braham (Ed.), *The psychological perspectives of the Holocaust and of its aftermath* (pp. 45-52). New York: Columbia University Press.

Norris, F.H. (1992). Epidemiology of trauma: Frequency and impact of different potentially traumatic events on different demographic groups. *Journal of Consulting and Clinical Psychology, 60,* 409-418.

Nurge, E. (Ed.). *The modern Sioux: Social systems and reservation culture.* Lincoln, NE: University of Nebraska Press.

Osgood, C.E., Suci, G.J., & Tannenbaum, P.H. (1978). *The measurement of meaning.* Urbana & Chicago: University of Illinois Press. (original work published 1957).

Powers, M. (1986). *Oglala women.* Chicago: University of Chicago Press.

Pribor, E.F., Yutzy, S.H., Dean, T., & Wetzel, R.D. (1993). Briquet's syndrome, dissociation, and abuse. *American Journal of Psychiatry, 150,* 1507-1511.

Resick, P.A. & Schnicke, M.K. (1992). Cognitive processing therapy for sexual assault victims. *Journal of Consulting and Clinical Psychology, 60*(5), 748-756.

Robin, R.W., Chester, B., & Goldman, D. (1996). Cumulative trauma and PTSD in American Indian communities. In Marsella, A.J., Friedman, M.J., Gerrity, E.T., & Scurfield, R.M. (Eds), *Ethnocultural aspects of Post-traumatic Stress Disorder.* Washington, DC: American Psychological Association, pp. 239-253.

Saxe, G.N., Chinman, G., Berkowitz, R., Hall, K., Lieberg, G., Schwartz, J., & van der Kolk, B.A. (1994). Somatization in patients with dissociative disorders. *American Journal of Psychiatry, 151,* 1329-1335.

Schonfeld, W.H., Verboncoeur, C.J., Fifer, S.K., Lipschutz, R.C., Lubeck, D.P., & Buesching, D.P. (1997). The functioning and well-being of patients with unrecognized anxiety disorders and major depressive disorder. *Journal of Affective Disorders, 43*(2), 105-119.

Shapiro, P.A. (1996). Psychiatric aspects of cardiovascular disease. *Psychiatric Clinics of North America, 19*(3), 613-629.

Shore, J. H., Manson, S. M., Bloom, J.D., Keepers, G., & Neligh, G. (1987). A pilot study of depression among American Indian patients with research diagnostic criteria. *American Indian and Alaska Native Mental Health Research, 1*(2), 4-15.

Sigal, J. & Weinfeld, M. (1989). *Trauma and rebirth: Intergenerational effects of the Holocaust.* New York: Praeger.

Silver, S. M. & Wilson, J. P. (1988). Native American healing and purification rituals for war stress. In John P. Wilson, Zev Harele, & Boaz Hahana (Eds.) *Human adaptation to extreme stress: From the Holocaust to Viet Nam* (pp. 337-355). New York: Plenum Press.

Tanner, H. (1982). *A history of all the dealings of the United States government with the Sioux.* Unpublished manuscript. Prepared for the Black Hills Land Claim by order of the United States Supreme Court, on file at the D'Arcy McNickle Center for the History of the American Indian, Newberry Library, Chicago.

Thomas, J.A. (1984). Race, color, and essential hypertension: A proposal for an international symposium. *Journal of the National Medical Association, 76*(4), 393-399.

Ursano, R.J., Grieger, T.A., & McCarroll, J.E. (1996). Prevention of post-traumatic stress: Consultation, training, and early treatment. In van der Kolk, B.A., McFarlane, A.C., & Weisaeth, L. (Eds.), *Traumatic stress: The effects of overwhelming experience on mind, body, and society.* New York: Guilford Press, pp. 441-462.

van der Kolk, B.A. (1996). The body keeps the score: Approaches to the psychobiology of Post-traumatic Stress Disorder. In van der Kolk, B.A., McFarlane, A.C., & Weisaeth, L. (Eds.), *Traumatic stress: The effects of overwhelming experience on mind, body, and society.* New York: Guilford Press, pp. 214-241.

van der Kolk, B.A., McFarlane, A.C., & van der Hart, O. (1996). A general approach to treatment of Post-traumatic Stress Disorder. In van der Kolk, B.A., McFarlane, A.C., & Weisaeth, L. (Eds.), *Traumatic stress: The effects of overwhelming experience on mind, body, and society.* New York: Guilford Press, pp. 417-440.

van der Kolk, B.A., Roth, S., Pelcovitz, D. & Mandel, F. (1993). *Complex PTSD: Results of the PTSD field trials for DSM-IV.* Washington, DC: American Psychiatric Association.

van der Kolk, B.A. (1987). *Psychological trauma.* Washington, DC: American Psychiatric Press.

Van Winkle, N.W. & May, P.A. (1993). An update on American Indian suicide in New Mexico, 1980-1987. *Human Organization, 52*(3), 304-315.

Weaver, H.N. (1996). Social work with American Indian youth using the orthogonal model of cultural identification. *Families in Society: The Journal of Contemporary Human Services, 77*(2), 98-107.

Weaver, H.N. & Brave Heart, M.Y.H. (1999). Examining two facets of American Indian identity: Exposure to other cultures and the influence of historical trauma. *Journal of Human Behavior in the Social Environment 2*(1/2), 19-33.

Welty, T.K. & Coulehan, J.L. (1993). Cardiovascular disease among American Indians and Alaska Natives. *Diabetes Care, 16*(1), 277-283.

Zitzow, D. & Desjarlait, F. (1994). A study of suicide attempts comparing adolescents to adults on a Northern Plains American Indian reservation. *American Indian and Alaska Native Mental Health Research, 4*(Mono), 35-69.

At What Cost? The Social Impact of American Indian Gaming

Thomas D. Peacock, EdD
Priscilla A. Day, MSW
Robert B. Peacock, MEd

SUMMARY. American Indian gaming has been called the "new buffalo." It has the potential to greatly influence cultural traditions on American Indian reservations. This study looks at the social impact that American Indian gaming is having on one reservation in northern Minnesota. Tribal members share strong feelings, both positive and negative, about the issue. Concerns about gaming include an increase in gambling abuse and addiction; a lack of appropriate child care; and concern that gaming is replacing traditional social activities. Some express concern that American Indian values are being replaced by materialism. Supporters of gaming point out that gaming provides tribal members with an opportunity to learn job skills and have gainful employment. Implications for social policy are given. *[Article copies available for a fee from The Haworth Document Delivery Service: 1-800-342-9678. E-mail address: getinfo@haworthpressinc.com]*

One of the most controversial issues in American Indian communities today is gambling. Some have called gaming the "new buffalo," touting it as something that could help to restore American Indians to their former pre-contact status. Studies have begun to be done looking at the economic impact of gaming on Indian communities and their surrounding environments but virtually no studies have looked at the social impact that gaming is having on these communities nor the potential long term impact on cultural traditions. This study is a first step in documenting the impact that the introduction of gaming has had on the residents of one reservation in northern Minnesota. Recommendations for tribal and mainstream policy makers are given.

This study uses a qualitative methodology to let American Indian community members describe in their own words the impact gaming has had in their lives and in the lives of other community members. Although only one community is represented here, their voices are important reminders that there is impact beyond economics that policy makers, both tribal and mainstream, should take into consideration when making decisions about American Indian gaming.

BACKGROUND

America has seen a large increase in legalized gambling in the past several decades. By 1997 gambling was legal in 48 out of 50 states and over 115 Indian tribes had class III gaming operations (video machines/table games and/or bingo) with 131 tribal/state compacts approved in 23 states. Approximately 80% of the adult population has participated in gambling (Lesieur & Rosenthal, 1991).

Gambling in Minnesota became a public business with the establishment of horse racing in 1982 and a state lottery in 1988 (Zitzow, 1996). Today, Minnesota residents spend almost $336 million on various forms of lottery and an additional $66 million on horse racing. Over $1.38 billion is being wagered on charitable gambling (Minnesota Indian Gaming Association, 1997). In addition to the various forms of state authorized gambling described above, Indian gaming is also available in the State of Minnesota. There are currently 11 Indian tribes involved in the operation of casinos in the state, offering approximately 12,900 slot machines and almost 500 table games (Minnesota Indian Gaming Association, 1997).

As legalized gambling in Minnesota has expanded so have gambling related problems. Specifically, problem gambling is identified as a behavior in which a person suffers some loss of control over his or her gambling, leading to negative consequences (Lesieur & Blume, 1987). More serious gambling problems are identified as pathological gambling behavior, which is typified as a chronic and progressive psychological disorder characterized by emotional dependence, loss of control and accompanying negative consequences in the gambler's school, work, social or family life (American Psychiatric Association, 1987). Studies indicate that between 4% and 6% of the adult population has a gambling problem (O'Brien, 1993). Other findings conducted with juveniles indicate that between 9% and 14% of the population are experiencing symptoms of problem gambling and between 4% and 7% meet the criteria for pathological gambling (Shaffer & Hall, 1994).

As gambling grows, greater attention is being directed to the public health risks that accompany it. A Nechi Institute study found that 60% of identified problem gamblers are former alcohol and drug users (Hodgson, 1994). Other literature also indicates a high degree of correlation between alcoholism and the potential for gambling addiction (Zitzow, 1996). Jacobs (1991) examined similarities between alcohol and gambling addiction, and expressed concern that the conditions and characteristics that predispose a person to alcohol misuse may also predispose them to problematic gambling. High rates of alcohol use and abuse among American Indians, as a group, have been well documented in numerous studies (Zitzow, 1996; Midwest Regional Center, 1988). Depression, poverty and unemployment within American Indian communities also appear to have the potential of increasing gambling problems, since they already appear to increase alcohol addictions. American Indian adolescents are at greater risk for problem gambling and the resultant problems associated with problem gambling (Peacock, Day, & Peacock, 1999).

Research literature on the social impact of gaming on individuals and communities, as well as the impact on tribal cultures, is virtually non-existent. This study broke new ground by exploring issues of gaming from a sociological and cultural perspective.

METHODS

The reservation participating in the study covers 2 counties with a resident Indian population of 5,800 of a total population of approximately 56,000 people. Within the reservation there are three separate and distinct villages with primarily American Indian residents. Two major population centers with populations over 10,000 are located on the Northwest and Southeast reservation boundaries outside the reservation. The reservation has one major interstate highway bisecting it and a nearby regional airport which handles commercial jet traffic. Both the small cities and the reservation are rural in nature and somewhat isolated from the rest of the state. Most of the land on the reservation is owned by the United States and controlled by the U.S. Forestry Service. The remaining lands are held in trust by the United States for the tribe or are privately owned.

Permission to conduct the study was obtained from the tribal council. Open-ended interviews of thirty (30) American Indian residents were done. Participants were selected by the authors using purposive (elders, educators, human service workers, reservation administrators, gender) sampling. Some informants chose a pseudonym for purposes of reporting out the data. Written assurances of anonymity were included in signed consent forms.

The data generated for the study came from in-depth phenomenological interviewing based on a method developed for a study of community colleges by Irving Seidman and Patrick Sullivan and later described by Seidman in *Interviewing as Qualitative Research* (1991). The theoretical underpinnings of this method stem from the phenomenologists in general and Alfred Schutz (1967) in particular. In this model, the researcher deems the experience of the participant with regard to the subject being studied as important in coming to an understanding of that subject. This interviewing strives to maximize the participant's rendering of that experience.

A series of three interviews provided enough time, privacy, and trust so that the participant could relate his or her experience, reflect on that experience, and to some extent, make sense of it. The study explored informants' perceptions of the issues involving casino gaming in their communities, and requested suggestions for reservation administrators and tribal council members on how they might resolve the issues. The first interview explored the informant's background and experiences with gaming. Interview two focused on the social, educational, economic and cultural impact of gaming. The final interview explored their suggestions to ameliorate the negative impact of gaming in reservation communities. The study design was approved by the University of Minnesota human subjects committee.

The research design is qualitative and uses Grounded Theory (Glaser & Strauss, 1967) as a way of studying the impact of gaming on the reservation. Grounded Theory relies on the constant comparative method, the joint coding and analysis of data using analytic induction (Bogdan & Bilken, 1982; Ely, 1991), and the premise that theory evolves from the data and is illustrated by examples from it. Because theory evolves from emerging data, there is no hypothesis at the inception of the research. Interview data was sorted into emerging themes and based on the juxtaposition of what the different informants said. Category codes based on themes are developed. The three open-ended tape recorded interviews with each informant are approximately one (1) hour each. Tapes of the completed interviews were transcribed as interviews were completed. The interview data was sorted and analyzed with the assistance of ETHNOGRAPH, a qualitative research software program.

In using informant quotes, we allowed ourselves to take out the repetitive comments and material that were extraneous to the topic being covered. We wove material from different parts of the three interviews when they were on the same topic. Then, we changed the tenses of verbs so the material from these different parts of the interview would work together. Most important, everything that is quoted is in the informants' own words, and we have committed ourselves to present them in a way that is in concert with the integrity of everything the informants said. Finally, we chose strong quotes which reflected the collective voices of the people interviewed in the study.

FINDINGS

There was little middle ground in the perceptions informants had toward gaming's impact on the social and cultural aspects of tribal life. Those who viewed the effects as negative focused on: a perception that gambling was replacing alcohol abuse as an addiction, with an accompanying neglect of family responsibilities caused by gambling addiction; a decrease in family and other community social activities as they are replaced by casino gambling as the dominant social activity; problems with child care as gamblers and casino workers alike are relying on young people to provide child care, or neglecting to provide child care altogether because extended family members are either working in casinos or gambling.

Conversely, some informants felt the new found presence of casinos resulted in a stronger and more positive collective consciousness, and increase in individual self-worth through gainful employment. Moreover, the presence of casinos on the reservation, and its draw of large numbers of non-Indian customers, was exposing many reservation residents and non-Indians to face to face contact for the first time. Many of these informants felt the increased interaction was positive for both non-Indians and Indians, as it served to break down mutually negative stereotypes the groups have of each other. Some felt this particularly benefitted many Indian residents whose exposure to non-Indians would help them live better in both worlds.

There was a deep sense from most informants that the presence of casino gaming was having yet undetermined effects on traditional tribal culture (values, beliefs, ways of being), that these effects were most probably negative and would become apparent in the near future. This almost took on a sense of foreboding about what the future would bring for traditional culture. Informants spoke of a decline in leveling (a sharing of material possessions based upon traditional values) with the increase in jobs, money and the rise in individual materialism. Conversely, others felt the increase in jobs and money associated with gaming was rebuilding both individual and communities identities, both which have long suffered from poverty, despair, and accompanying social ills.

The Social Impact of Casino Gaming

By far the most positive finding is that gaming has provided much needed employment on the reservation, and nothing works better to improve both the collective consciousness and individual self-worth than steady employment at a livable wage.

> It's given some people jobs. And income where they've never had income before. You know, they've been able to hold these jobs. Now they work. They're different people. So in that aspect it's been good.

While decent jobs may lead to an increased sense of self-worth for some, the presence of a casino can lead to problems. Alcohol addiction has been a pervasive problem in some American Indian communities. Many reservations have developed successful prevention and out/inpatient treatment programs to deal with problems of alcoholism in their communities. Progress in dealing with alcoholism and its accompanying social ills has been remarkable in the past several decades.

But addictive behavior, be it alcoholism, other chemicals, or gambling, all offer similar temporary euphoria in the brain's pleasure centers (Zitzow, 1996). Many of the informants noted that as some Indian people who are addicted to alcohol successfully complete treatment programs and begin to make healthy life choices, some exchange one addiction with another, gambling. This collective sense was captured by one informant.

From what I can see that a lot of people are involved in gaming in some way. One of the things that they do is play bingo. People that before were heavy drinkers or problem drinkers and have quit that and are gambling instead. And, in other ways, I don't know if it's really has had a social [impact], in a sense that it's, like the powwows and that. There's a lot of people that are involved in powwows, activities of that kind and go to them. For some people it has affected them. They're more apt to spend time with people at bingo. "Are you going to the casino? Are you going to play bingo? I'll go with you." Or, "If you want, come with me." For some people it's that activity some of the time. Well, for some people, it gets them out to do things, gives them an activity. And for some people, it becomes a habit. That's all they like. They rush through their normal everyday activities so they can have a chance to attend bingo sessions or sometimes they need it. And for other people, it something to do on occasion, you know, as a treat. A lot were serious drinkers in the past, [one] an alcoholic who has been sober for over the last fourteen years, is in the casinos now. There's people that I used to hang out with, drink with, they became sober. [Now] they're replacing one thing with the other–like we used to drink on weekends, and in place of that activity, now they're going to go into casinos. It's about equal to the amount of time that they spent drinking. It's out of control for some.

Georgiana

Related to and often accompanying the issue of adult gambling addiction is the fact that those who can least afford it are sometimes the most affected by it. Alan is an American Indian school social work aide in a reservation public school, who spoke passionately about the issue:

> Parents, even older students, here that really can't afford to due to a large family or the economics of it go in there [casino] to gamble. Especially with the recipients for AFDC [Aid to Families of Dependent Children], you know. That's a big issue here.

The growth of casino gaming has sometimes taxed limited child care opportunities. With large numbers of people (particularly many women entering the labor market for the first time) as well as a perceived increase in adult addictive gambling behavior, the burden of child care has sometimes fallen on the shoulders of siblings, as well as neighborhood teens seeking babysitting jobs. Kathy, a former foster care worker, spoke for many of the informants.

> I feel like a lot of them [children] are left alone to be with no supervision. I just see that a lot of children are being just left to use their own judgment as to what to do with their time. And I have seen in my own career where I've worked as a foster licensing person and I saw where foster children are put in, in homes where gambling was a priority and the children have begun to sniff gas and use other substances. There was a lot of bizarre behavior because the children were being left while the adults were away at bingo. People that are involved with bingo, it's a lot like the cycle of alcoholism. Where that's the first priority. Sometimes it's just up to the children to decide what they're going to do with themselves.

Reservation communities are sometimes typified by sharp racial dividing lines, with Indians and non-Indians living together in close proximity but rarely interacting. As a result of this, these communities have developed separate economic, social and political systems. It is not unusual to see primarily Indian bowling, softball and basketball leagues exist in these communities, playing against their non-Indian neighbors only at occasional tournaments. Pow-wows and other cultural events are attended by few non-Indians. Most Indians work for the tribal government or at federal (Bureau of Indian Affairs or Indian Public Health Service) jobs. With the advent of casino gambling and its strong attraction to all segments of the community, Indian and non-Indian alike, the two communities were interacting on a regular basis for the first time. This was pointed out by Billy Jo, a tribal education worker, who felt this interaction was having a positive effect on both communities by helping break down old stereotypes:

> I think that just by having the casino here it's something that residents can be proud of. It brings people in. I think that it's a plus because [of] where it's located at and the powwow that goes on sometimes. Non-Indians come for their sole purpose of gambling, out of curiosity maybe wander over to the powwow grounds and be able to learn more about us and just to become aware of that we [are], of who we are, and get a taste of what we're about. And maybe it may squash some of the kind of stereotypes they may have or say, they, well, maybe that's not what I thought, how I thought it was going to be. Some people have never been on a reservation before, and having casinos there, it's bringing people in.

Many informants noticed a decline in the numbers of people partaking in other social activities with the growth in casino gaming, as gambling quickly became the dominant social activity in the community. Carolyn, an educator, spoke for many of the informants in this regard.

> You see people that had previously been doing other things, you know, maybe in the community, aren't now. You see them more out to the casinos. People that I'd known before that have been involved like in, oh, like their clubs in downtown, like VFW and stuff like that. You see those are decreasing, where the people are out doing, they are out gambling rather than attending functions they previously attended. Lot of the church functions, too, they're down. I know my mother has mentioned many times that their women's groups are not quite as active as they used to be.

The Effects of Gaming on Tribal Culture

One aspect of how gaming may alter tribal culture was echoed by Mike, a counselor in the tribal school, as tribes move away from a traditional society based on leveling to one of individual materialism. He captured the sentiment of many of those interviewed.

> I think anytime you think of Indian gaming, you think of money. And, you know that's contrary to a lot of Indian culture, [where]

you place the emphasis on bucks and dollars and making it rich. Putting everything in value in dollars, and it's very contrary to Indian culture. Certainly what we have to look at the same time that, you know, is that money means survival in this day and age. I think it's a blending, a blending that just takes place, it's–a blending when you're having to work for a living. And I think, again, it's like anything else, it's when you abuse it, then it develops into abuse. [When] gaming is abused and children go without food, without shelter, I think it goes against all Indian values. If it affects the culture in some way, it affects the spirituality.

A core of informants felt the advent of casino gaming at this point was having an undetermined effect on traditional Indian culture. This almost took on a sense of foreboding in some, who felt the long-term impact on tribal culture was going to be negative, but couldn't put a finger on what these effects might be. Others felt the effects were positive, as the tribal council was putting more resources into the pow-wows. Still others felt it was giving Indian people a stronger and more positive sense of identity.

I think it's made Indian people feel more empowered, in a sense. You know, because they have the casinos. I think they feel like they possibly can do more, whether it's good or bad. If it's just for good then, I think it's made them more visible.

Carolyn

She went on to say that young people who were raised in their traditional ways should not be affected by the modern casino industry. But she wasn't sure, and her sentiment captured the collective wondering of many of those interviewed.

I really don't know how to say it affects their culture because if they're [traditional], it's more ingrained in them, it's something you shouldn't lose. I really don't know if it is affecting their culture or not. I really don't know. I would say yes [it is], in the sense that if they are becoming addicted and are going all the time, why, they're not keeping in mind their [spirituality]. I think they're not quite as involved in [spirituality/traditional ways] as they possibly might have been.

IMPLICATIONS

American Indian gaming provokes strong sentiment whether on the reservation or off. As this study found, there are both positive and negative social impacts for reservations and their members. This impact obviously spills over into non-Indian communities. American Indian gaming has brought Indian and non-Indian cultures colliding together socially and economically.

The implications for social policy are numerous. Social policy makers, whether tribal or mainstream, could work to counter some of the negative influences of gaming. This could be done by mandating a redistribution of a percentage of gaming income towards gambling abuse prevention and treatment programs; funding non-gaming family and community activities–especially those with a focus on traditional American Indian culture; and by the development of appropriate child care.

Additionally, mandated research that is culturally appropriate needs to be sponsored by tribal groups to focus on the social impact of gaming in reservation communities with special attention paid to the potential long term effects on American Indian culture and traditions. Is Indian gaming the "new buffalo" or will it erode traditional American Indian culture further? Only time will tell.

REFERENCES

American Psychiatric Association. (1987). *Diagnostic and statistical manual of mental disorders* (3rd edition, revised DSM-III-R). Washington, DC: American Psychiatric Association.

Bogdan, R.C., & Bilken, S.K. (1982). *Qualitative research for education: An introduction in theory and methods.* Needham Heights, MA: Allyn and Bacon.

Ely, M. (1991). *Doing qualitative research: Circles within circles.* Bristol, PA: Falmer Press.

Glaser, A., & Strauss, B. (1967). *The discovery of grounded theory.* New York: Aldine.

Hodgson, M. (1995). *Spirit of bingo land.* Edmonton, Alberta: Nechi Institute of Alcohol and Drug Education.

Jacobs, D. (1991). Teenage gambling in America. *Treatment Center Magazine, 43.*

Lesieur, H., & Blume, S. (1987). The south oaks gambling screen (SOGS): A new instrument for the identification of pathological gamblers. *American Journal of Psychiatry, 144* (9), 1184-1188.

Midwest Regional Center. (1988). Midwest study of ethnic difference regarding alcohol and other substance abuse. Chicago: U.S. Department of Education.

Miller Cleary, L. & Peacock, T. (1998). *Collected wisdom: American Indian education.* Needham Heights, MA: Allyn and Bacon.

Minnesota Indian Gaming Association. (1997). Economic benefits of Indian gaming in the state of Minnesota. Minneapolis: MIGA.

O'Brien, J. (1993). Why gamblers can't walk away from the table. *Your Health*, p. 13.

Peacock, R., Day, P., & Peacock, T. (1999). Adolescent gaming on a Great Lakes Indian reservation. *Journal of Human Behavior in the Social Environment, 2* (1/2) 5-17.

Schultz, A. (1967). *The phenomenology of the social world.* Evanston, IL: Northwestern University Press.

Seidman, I.E. (1991). *Interviewing as qualitative research.* New York: Teachers College Press.

Shaffer, H., & Hall, M. (1994). Estimating the prevalence of adolescent gambling disorders: A quantitative synthesis and guide toward standard gambling nomenclature. Boston: Harvard Medical School.

Zitzow, D. (1996). A comparative study of problematic gambling behaviors between American Indian and non-Indian adolescents within and near a northern plains reservation. *American Indian and Alaskan Native Mental Health Research, 7* (2) 14-26.

Protecting the Future of Indigenous Children and Nations: An Examination of the Indian Child Welfare Act

Hilary N. Weaver, DSW
Barry J. White, MA

SUMMARY. The Indian Child Welfare Act is a landmark piece of legislation, passed in response to a long history of Native American children being alienated from their families and communities. The Act has far reaching implications for social workers and human service professionals who have any involvement with Native American children or families. Still, many professionals are either unaware of the Act all together or do not know how to effectively implement its provisions in their practice. This lack of awareness and other factors such as inadequate funding have meant that the Act has never realized its full potential to reduce the number of children in out-of-home care. In order to increase awareness about the Act and to make its implementation in day to day social services more practical, this article provides background information on the factors leading to the Act, information on the law itself, and recommendations for practitioners, administrators, and students in the human services. *[Article copies available for a fee from The Haworth Document Delivery Service: 1-800-342-9678. E-mail address: getinfo@haworthpressinc.com]*

"There is no resource more vital to the continued existence and integrity of Indian tribes than their children" (P.L. 95-608, Section 2

(3)). The Indian Child Welfare Act of 1978 (ICWA) is a landmark piece of legislation, passed in response to a long history of Native American children being alienated from their families and communities. The Act has far reaching implications for social workers and human service professionals who have any involvement with Native American children or families. Still, many professionals are either unaware of the Act all together or do not know how to effectively implement its provisions in their practice. This lack of awareness and other factors such as inadequate funding have meant that the Act has never realized its full potential to reduce the number of children in out-of-home care.

In order to increase awareness about the Act and to make its implementation in day to day social services more practical, this article provides background information on the factors leading to the Act and the law itself. Parts of the discussion are illustrated with details of how ICWA functions within the state of New York. Although the details given are specific to one area of the country, this examination provides useful comparisons for other regions. Finally, recommendations are offered concerning proper implementation of ICWA by practitioners, administrators, and students in the human services.

BACKGROUND: FACTORS LEADING TO ICWA

The reasons for the federal law as stated in the Act itself include recognition that "an alarmingly high percentage of Indian families are broken up by the removal, often unwarranted, of their children from them by nontribal public and private agencies and that an alarmingly high percentage of such children are placed in non-Indian foster and adoptive homes and institutions" (P.L. 95-608, Section 2(4)). The policy of separating Native children from their families began with the boarding schools around the time of the American Civil War (Johnson, 1981). These schools, frequently long distances from reservations, were designed to assimilate Native American children into the dominant society. Prior to the passage of ICWA, between 25 and 35% of all Native American children were separated from their families and 85% of these were placed in non-Native substitute care (Dorsay, 1984; Mannes, 1995). Native American children experienced a placement rate between 5 and 25 times higher than that of their non-Native peers (U.S. Senate Select Committee on Indian Affairs, 1977). Native

American children tended to remain in foster care longer and be moved from one foster home to another more frequently than White children (Barsh, 1996). Native American children raised away from their families and communities are often left with little or none of their cultural heritage (Mannes, 1995) and often experience significant social problems which are rooted in a sense of abandonment and ethnic confusion (Barsh, 1996; U.S. Senate Select Committee on Indian Affairs, 1977; 1988).

Ignorance and cultural misunderstandings have frequently led to inappropriate handling of Native American cases in child welfare proceedings. Resources in Native American communities often go unrecognized (Blanchard & Barsh, 1980). Problematic interactions go beyond individual encounters and are sometimes institutionalized in policies or laws. "Congress found that frequent unnecessary removals of Indian children had been the result of *professional and judicial attitudes* towards Indians, *state judicial procedures*, and the design and accessibility of *federal child welfare programs*" (Barsh, 1996, 236-237; italics in original).

Licensing standards for foster homes frequently exclude Native families on the basis of income levels and physical features of the home. Often state licensing standards for foster homes are based on the assumption that material comfort is a prerequisite to adequate nurturing of children (Barsh, 1996). There is no reason to believe that the poverty which many Native American families face renders them unfit parents or that some reason exists why the cases of child neglect which do exist cannot be dealt with satisfactorily within Native American communities rather than by state intervention (U.S. Senate Select Committee on Indian Affairs, 1977).

When developing the Indian Child Welfare Act, one of the primary goals of Congress was to set strict procedural limitations on state and private child welfare agencies (Barsh, 1996). In a clear statement made by Senator Abourezk, Chairman of the U.S. Senate Committee on Indian Affairs which heard testimony prior to the passage of ICWA, he indicted non-Native social service agencies for their racism and operational premise that most Indian children would really be better off growing up non-Indian. "The Federal Government for its part has been conspicuous by its lack of action. It has chosen to allow these agencies to strike at the heart of Indian communities by literally stealing Indian children ... It has been called cultural genocide" (U.S. Senate Select Committee on Indian Affairs, 1977, 2).

THE CONTEXT AND CONTENT OF ICWA

The Indian Child Welfare Act of 1978 was more than ten years in the making. For years Native people expressed concerns about the loss of their children. In 1968 in response to these concerns the Association on American Indian Affairs conducted a survey of custody problems in Native American communities. This was followed in 1974 by the first Congressional hearing on this matter (Dorsay, 1984; Mannes, 1995). In 1976 the third annual convention of the National Congress of American Indians representing 130 Native nations unanimously supported a draft of the major provisions which later became ICWA (U.S. Senate Select Committee on Indian Affairs, 1977). In the 1977 Senate hearings and the 1978 House of Representatives hearings many Native people including representatives from over 30 Native nations and organizations spoke and/or submitted written statements in favor of the bill and recommended changes which would clarify or strengthen certain parts. Many non-Native representatives of organizations and states testified or submitted written statements in support of ICWA (U.S. Senate Select Committee on Indian Affairs, 1977).

While many of the concerns expressed about the bill involved refining and clarifying language, one substantive concern was echoed time and time again. That concern was over how "Indian child" was defined within the legislation and therefore in which cases the law would be applied. For purposes of the Act, "Indian child" is defined as "any unmarried person who is under age eighteen and is either (a) a member of an Indian tribe or (b) is eligible for membership in an Indian tribe and is the biological child of a member of an Indian tribe" (P.L. 95-608).

This concern has been debated in Congressional hearings since the passage of ICWA (U.S. Senate Select Committee on Indian Affairs, 1980; 1984; 1988; 1996) and has also been debated in numerous legal cases. (See "Notes of decisions," 25 U.S.C.A., chapter 21, section 19). The definition of "Indian child" excludes many Native American children who do not meet enrollment requirements for their particular nations. Enrollment requirements, qualifications for citizenship in a Native nation, are often based on factors such as blood quantum or descent from a person listed on the tribal census on a given date. Members of Native nations which are not federally recognized by the United States and members of Canadian nations are not covered under ICWA (Barsh, 1996; Dorsay, 1984). It is unclear whether the provisions apply to some Alaskan Natives (Barsh, 1996; Dorsay, 1984). Although many Native Americans see the definition of Indian child as being too narrow and excluding many who could benefit from the protection of the Act, some other people, most notably adoption organizations and attorneys, see the definition as too inclusive (Bakeis, 1996).

The Act became law November 8th, 1978 and its jurisdictional provisions took effect in May of 1979 (U.S. Senate Select Committee on Indian Affairs, 1980). The Act is first and foremost a statement about jurisdiction in custody proceedings. A Native American nation has a right to conduct or be involved in any custody proceeding involving a child of that nation. The Act defines child custody proceedings to include foster care placements, pre-adoptive placements, adoption, or termination of parental rights (American Indian Law Center, 1986; Barsh, 1996; Dorsay, 1984). Custody proceedings as part of a divorce are not covered. ICWA does not affect the power of states to intervene in Native American homes as a preventive measure or to remove Native children on the grounds of juvenile delinquency (Barsh, 1996; Dorsay, 1984).

Essentially ICWA provides seven major procedural safeguards when Native children are involved in custody proceedings: (1) exclusive tribal jurisdiction over children who live on reservations except where federal law already designated jurisdiction to the state, (2) authorization for Native nations to petition for previously lost jurisdiction, (3) the power for both parents and the Native nations to intervene in state proceedings involving Native children, (4) application of higher standards of proof when Native American children are involved in state initiated custody proceedings, (5) preference for placement with Native families and communities when state agencies place Native American children in substitute care, (6) informed consent must be demonstrated by Native parents in placement or adoption proceedings and they have an extended period in which to revoke consent, and (7) access to state records for Native nations and parents (Barsh, 1996).

The best interest of the child is frequently cited as the standard used in child welfare cases but it was not clearly defined by any statute until ICWA. ICWA clearly indicates that cultural continuity is in the best interest of the child. The fundamental concept behind ICWA is that protecting the cultural identity of Native American children will enable them to become well adjusted adults and will help preserve the cultural continuity and integrity of Native nations (Blanchard & Barsh, 1980; Dorsay, 1984).

IMPLEMENTATION

While many people and organizations have high praise for the intent of ICWA there is also concern that the effectiveness of the Act is limited by inconsistencies and ambiguities in the law itself (Barsh, 1996). Although questions of the constitutionality of ICWA have been raised since before its passage (U.S. House of Representatives Subcommittee on Indian Affairs and Public Lands, 1981), challenges to the Act on this basis have thus far been unsuccessful (Barsh, 1996).

Implementation of ICWA varies tremendously across the country. Some Native nations and organizations cite growing cooperation between states and tribes as a positive effect of ICWA although there is still room for improvement (U.S. Senate Select Committee on Indian Affairs, 1984). Some states passed legislation with similar intent and provisions to ICWA. The places which have implemented ICWA with the most success tend to have state laws which reinforce it (U.S. Senate Select Committee on Indian Affairs, 1988).

A lack of infrastructure to support the intent of ICWA has led to problems in its implementation. In response to ICWA, tribal governments were faced with the daunting task of developing or enhancing social and legal services necessary to respond to the needs of Native children involved in custody proceedings (Ware, Dobrec, Rosenthal, & Wedel, 1992). Many Native American nations enacted or expanded existing child welfare services. Most staff learned their jobs through on the job training (Wares, Wedel, Rosenthal, & Dobrec, 1994), however, it is interesting to note that according to a 1986 evaluation of ICWA, tribally run programs are more likely than state programs to employ BSW and MSW staff to provide child welfare services (U.S. Senate Select Committee on Indian Affairs, 1986).

The first systematic nationwide study of the effects of ICWA was commissioned by the Administration for Children, Youth and Families and the Bureau of Indian Affairs in 1986. This study found that the rate of Native American children in substitute care was still 3.6 times the rate for non-Native children and in fact the number of Native children in care had risen from about 7,200 in the early 1980s to 9,005 in 1986 in spite of the fact that there was a decrease in the number of children of all races in substitute care during that timeframe (U.S. Senate Select Committee on Indian Affairs, 1988). In 1986, 63% of Native children in foster care were in homes with at least one Indian parent. The study found that public program case records indicated that in 65-70% of the cases, parents had been notified of proceedings and tribes had been notified in 80% of the cases. In most cases states willingly transferred jurisdiction of cases to tribes; however, in some cases, requests were denied because of socioeconomic conditions on reservations or the perceived inadequacies of tribal social services or judicial systems. This is clearly a violation of the BIA's *Guidelines for State Courts* for implementing ICWA. In spite of the fact that ICWA requires active preventive efforts be made prior to removal, preventive efforts were found to have taken place in only 41% of the cases reviewed (U.S. Senate Select Committee on Indian Affairs, 1988). Federal efforts to monitor and enforce compliance are limited and in some areas noncompliance is quite pronounced (U.S. Senate Select Committee on Indian Affairs, 1984; 1988).

Some state social welfare agencies and courts have been known to ignore the jurisdiction of Native nations over reservation children (Barsh, 1996). Cases have been documented in which state courts failed to transfer jurisdiction based on factors such as lack of confidence in the tribe to handle the matter, a child not having the intellectual capacity to benefit from upbringing in a tribal setting (even though intelligence had never been evaluated), no appropriate Native American families available to raise the child (even though availability had been documented) or based on the fact that a child had lived half her life outside of a Native community and it would be a hardship to transport a State's witness to a tribal court (U.S. Senate Select Committee on Indian Affairs, 1984). These actions by state social welfare agencies and courts are clearly in violation of ICWA and continue to perpetuate the problems which ICWA was designed to address.

MacEachron, Gustavsson, Cross, and Lewis (1996) used data from existing surveys to determine the effect of ICWA. They found that by

1986 the average state adoption rate of Native children had dropped, the average state foster care placement rate had dropped, and the discrepancy between Native and non-Native adoption rates decreased. While MacEachron and colleagues (1986) offer tentative indications that foster care and adoption rates for Native children decreased substantially between 1975 and 1986, other authors indicate that these numbers did not in fact decrease but substitute care shifted from a state to a tribal or Native social service organization responsibility (Mannes, 1995; Ware, Dobrec, Rosenthal, & Wedel, 1992). During this timeframe overall out-of-home placement rates were declining.

Lack of funding has always been a major obstacle to implementation. Funding of tribal family support and child welfare programs and the manner in which the BIA allocated funds was identified as a problem immediately (Barsh, 1996; U.S. Senate Select Committee on Indian Affairs, 1980; 1984). Unclear and contradictory granting requirements and inefficient notification procedures affected funding for many Native nations and organizations (U.S. Senate Select Committee on Indian Affairs, 1980). Lack of resources led to tribes not accepting jurisdiction in some cases and not assuming custody in others. The Association of American Indian and Alaska Native Social Workers called for more adequate funding and pointed out the failure of the BIA to set in place appropriate recording mechanisms. "The lack of adequate reporting systems together with on again, off again funding patterns directly undermine the developmental efforts of tribal and Indian organizational programs and severely curtail our opportunity to develop a stable knowledge base of Indian social services practice and theory" (U.S. Senate Select Committee on Indian Affairs, 1984, 100).

Funding continues to be a problem to this day. In 1997, all off reservation Native organizations with child welfare programs were notified that ICWA funds would no longer be available (J. Knapp, Executive Director of Native American Community Services of Erie and Niagara Counties, personal communication, August 13, 1997). Faced with this cutback many agencies are forced to severely reduce or eliminate their child welfare services.

Other concerns mentioned repeatedly were problems with communication and notification. In part, the problems in communication may be related to the failure of service agencies to identify and track Native American clients (U.S. Senate Select Committee on Indian Affairs, 1984). There is also a problem with judges, attorneys, social workers, and other agency personnel being unaware of the Act (Kessel & Robbins, 1984; U.S. Senate Select Committee on Indian Affairs, 1984). In 1988 the Senate held hearings regarding proposed amendments to ICWA. While noting strong support for the basic concept of the Act some changes were deemed necessary. Many of the concerns raised in the 1984 hearings were stated again in the testimony of 1988 including concerns about funding, concerns about placing Native children in non-Native homes, the need for training, inadequate coordination between the Department of the Interior and the Department of Health and Human Services, inconsistency in cooperative agreements between states and tribes, and state courts making different decisions about implementing the provisions of the Act which leads to uncertainties in interpretation and inadequate notification. Additionally, much of the discussion of the 1988 hearings continued to center around whether to broaden the definition of "Indian child" but in the end the definition remained the same (U.S. Senate Select Committee on Indian Affairs, 1988).

In 1996 a proposed amendment to ICWA known as Title III of the Adoption, Promotion and Stability Act sought to limit the applicability of ICWA in cases where the parents do not maintain tribal affiliations (U.S. Senate Select Committee on Indian Affairs, 1996). While the Senate did not pass this amendment, changes which would weaken the effect of ICWA are proposed regularly.

ICWA IN NEW YORK STATE: BACKGROUND AND IMPLEMENTATION

The Native American nations indigenous to the area now known as New York State entered into agreements which preserved their legal and sovereign rights throughout the historical periods of exploration, colonization, and development of the United States. The Native nations always maintained a level of sovereignty which would not abrogate traditional rights. Treaties guaranteed services, regulated trade and commerce, and established land boundaries for coming generations of unborn Native people.

New York State has continuously attempted to promote a positive relationship with Native American governments through a series of agreements. In one such early agreement shortly after the Civil War, New York State created a post for an Indian agent to oversee social service programs within the state. The role of Indian Agent evolved into an office known as the New York State Bureau of Indian Services.

Placement and adoption services were centralized in the Bureau of Indian Services in the mid-1800s. This arrangement continued until 1957 for all Native American Nations recognized by the State of New York. During the last 40 years the office has maintained an overseeing role with peripheral involvement in direct services. The office maintains its working relationship today through the partnership of its Native American administrator with the eight Native American Nations who receive technical assistance and supportive services from the Bureau. The federal government, Bureau of Indian Affairs (BIA), works with the New York State Bureau in an effort to promote services and policies it establishes for federally recognized Native American nations. Federally recognized Native nations are those that the U.S. government acknowledges and with which it continues to have some sort of relationship. This includes six of the eight Native nations within the boundaries of New York State.

When ICWA was passed Native American human service workers began to network and create linkages with county agencies and service providers. The grassroots network that developed among Native American human service workers led to a gradual improvement of services, referrals, and placement under the ICWA. The New York State Indian Services Bureau promoted local district dialogue about the Act to encourage coordination of services with adjacent Native American Nations.

The Legal Division of the New York State Department of Social Services (NYSDSS) and the Bureau of Indian Services worked closely to develop regulations to implement the Indian Child Welfare Act within the State of New York. The result was an amendment to the New York State Family Court Act and the New York State Social Services Law which brought them into compliance with ICWA in terms of foster care and adoption of Native American children in New York State. The administrator of the Bureau of Indian Services developed plans to promote education about the law within NYSDSS and in Native American communities. The New York legislation became effective in the spring of 1987. The state extended the Indian Child Welfare Act, full faith and credit, to all Native American nations it recognizes, thereby extending protection to two Native nations recognized by the state but not the federal government. In 1993, the St.

Regis Mohawk Nation, located near Messina, New York, entered into the first ICWA tribal/state agreement with the New York State Department of Social Services. While such laws and agreements are promising, there are many counties in New York State that have not fully implemented these provisions. Until there is full compliance with the law, out-of-home placement rates for Native American children are likely to remain stable.

Native American urban agencies developed wide networks in Buffalo, Syracuse, Rochester, and New York, New York in an effort to educate local districts and agencies about ICWA. For example, Native American Community Services of Erie and Niagara counties (based in Buffalo, New York) conducted meetings with the local district commissioner in Erie County which resulted in a working relationship between the agency and the county on behalf of Native families impacted by ICWA.

OVERCOMING ROADBLOCKS TO IMPLEMENTATION: THE NEED FOR TRAINING

In order for ICWA to be fully implemented a key national issue that must be addressed is training. Training is needed for both tribal and state child welfare workers (Kessel & Robbins, 1984). Non-Native practitioners who work near reservations are often the first to ask for informational sessions on ICWA. Native American social workers are frequently placed in the position of "expert" by non-Native agencies who want to implement ICWA effectively. In addition to the rules and regulations of the law, the audience might also have a desire to know more about the local Native American way of life. Urban based Native American populations often saw the need for training on ICWA or culture diversity. The process of developing Native American training, marketing the curriculum and promoting the event might be overwhelming to a struggling Native child welfare program.

In New York State the Department of Social Services (NYSDSS) and Buffalo State College provide continuing education opportunities and training on a variety of social services topics (New York State Child Welfare Training Institute, 1992). In 1985, NYSDSS and Buffalo State College implemented training in cultural diversity. This three day training program includes one section on the Native American family and ICWA. The course is offered to a statewide audience of practitioners from public and voluntary agencies. The curriculum provides a multicultural approach to understanding service delivery issues for African American, Hispanic/Latino, Asian and Native American families. Training was also developed which is targeted toward the family court system, tribal judges, service providers from local districts, and the Native American social work community. This training increased awareness of ICWA and stimulated dialogue about tribal/state agreements. The general diversity training brought awareness and attention to a statewide audience who otherwise would not have been aware that a law exists that protects the rights of Native American children and nations.

In testimony given to Congress on the status of ICWA, the president of the Association of American Indian and Alaska Native Social Workers stated that the training needs of Native American nations and organizations have been completely neglected (U.S. Senate Select Committee on Indian Affairs, 1984). A survey done by this organization found that in ICWA matters social workers were required to function as paralegals. In a statement made by the President of the Oklahoma Indian Child Welfare Association, "We need to give the social workers the training they need, and they need to know when they are functioning as a social workers (sic) and they need to know when they are having to function as a paralegal . . . It is too heavy a burden without proper training. You certainly would not go out and try to repair your automobile with a screwdriver, and that is what we are trying to ask these social workers to do. We are asking them to have knowledge that is far beyond anything they have been trained or educated to do, and we are not going to have proper implementation until that training is a reality" (U.S. Senate Select Committee on Indian Affairs, 1984, 107).

In a survey of administrators of tribally based ICWA programs, 86% reported a line in their budget devoted to training. Sixty-eight percent attended state or regional workshops on ICWA, 52% attended national ICWA conferences, 42% attended national conferences which were not specific to ICWA, and 15% reported receiving other outside training (Wares et al., 1994). In spite of these workshops, survey respondents expressed concern about limited training on the job (Wares et al., 1994).

Tribal governments must pay more attention to the training needs of the administrators of ICWA programs (Wares et al., 1994). The first tribal/state agreement in New York State resulted in training of systems administrators, division heads, and program managers on cultural issues in working with Native American nations. Additional technical assistance for Native American nations was made available through the New York State Department of Social Services' Bureau of Indian Services and Buffalo State College (J. Wrightsman, Training Director, Center for Development of Human Services, personal communication, 9/9/97). In December 1996, a statewide teleconference was conducted to promote ICWA and to stimulate cross cultural understanding in service issues for Native American families (New York State Department of Social Services & State University of New York Research Foundation: Buffalo State College, 1996).

Some schools of social work have responded to the need for ICWA training. The University of Washington has developed a curriculum for both Native and non-Native child welfare personnel employed by the state and Native nations to deliver appropriate services. Likewise, Arizona State University has developed a curriculum for the White Mountain Apache to use in training their child protective services staff in a way which reflects their own cultural values (Wares et al., 1994).

Although there are still many complaints that lack of training in the provisions of ICWA has been a major hinderance in its implementation, some detailed training programs have been developed. The National Judicial College which is affiliated with the American Bar Association developed a training manual for judges and judicial educators. The training as they have developed it can be delivered in time slots of between two hours and two days and comes complete with an instructional outline and a self administered test with answers and case examples. The major points covered in this training are the legal basis and policy of ICWA, provisions of the Act, defining who is an Indian child under ICWA, procedural requirements for state courts, determining jurisdiction, placement standards, and practical skills in applying ICWA (Steele, 1995).

Conferences have been held which focus on ICWA in the hopes of promoting a better understanding and more thorough implementation of the Act. One such conference held at the American Indian Studies Center in Los Angeles had workshops which focused on how ICWA interacts with Public Law 280 (a 1953 law which allows states to have jurisdiction on Indian reservations), ICWA procedures and jurisdiction, and analysis of legal cases. Workshops also looked at cultural sensitivity, special needs children, and the long term effects of substitute care (Johnson, 1990).

CONCLUSION

ICWA is an important law which seeks to address a long history of Native American children being alienated from their parents and communities. While virtually everyone agrees that the intention of the Act is good, there is also consensus that it has not lived up to its potential because of problems in implementation. The following are recommendations which the authors believe would help substantially in implementing the spirit of the law.

Recommendations for Administrators and Politicians

1. Adequate funding must be available for Native nations and off reservation programs to deliver child welfare services.
2. States should pass their own laws which support ICWA and extend provisions to state recognized nations.
3. Agencies should embrace an inclusive definition of "Indian child." Whenever a Native child's nation can be identified, the agency policy should require notification of the relevant Native nation even if the child is not currently enrolled or the nation federally recognized.
4. Federal monitoring and enforcement of the Act must be improved.
5. Agency administrators and boards must encourage a climate of respect for ICWA both within their agencies and in the larger social service community.
6. Training must be provided for human service personnel, both Native and non-Native, on cultural issues. This training must include content on Native Americans. Training specific to the Indian Child Welfare Act must also be available to all human service workers.

Recommendations for Practitioners and Students in the Human Services

1. Practitioners should participate in continuing education or in-service training on cultural issues which includes content on Na-

tive American cultures and is delivered by Native American trainers.
2. Practitioners in social service agencies need continual training on how to implement the Indian Child Welfare Act in their practice.
3. Students in the human services should take at least one course which includes content on cultural diversity.
4. Practitioners must gather information about a client's ethnic background as part of a standard assessment.

The recommendations listed above are meant to serve as a guide to enhance the implementation of ICWA. ICWA is a unique policy which is grounded in values which embrace the well-being of the group as well as the well-being of the individual. In fact, in many Native American customs the two are synonymous; you cannot have a healthy nation without healthy individuals and vice versa. While few would dispute the applicability of this last sentence to any cultural group, it is clear that there is a strong White, middle-class, American value placed on individual freedom which continues to influence many other policies related to the well-being of children. In this sense, ICWA will always face cultural obstacles to implementation.

It is crucial that human service providers understand and do their best to implement the provisions of ICWA. The Act's spirit and intentions must be fulfilled. At stake is the well-being of Native American children, families, communities, nations, and in fact our very existence.

REFERENCES

American Indian Law Center (1986). *Indian Family Law and Child Welfare.* Albuquerque: American Indian Law Center.

Bakeis, C.D. (1996). The Indian Child Welfare Act of 1978: Violating personal rights for the sake of the tribe. *Notre Dame Journal of Law, Ethics and Public Policy, 10*(2), 543-586.

Barsh, R.L. (1996). The Indian Child Welfare Act of 1978: A critical analysis. In J.R. Wunder: *Recent Legal Issues for American Indians, 1968 to the Present.* New York: Garland Publishing. 219-268.

Johnson, B.B. (1981). The Indian Child Welfare Act of 1978: Implications for practice. *Child Welfare, 60*(7), 435-446.

Johnson, T.R. (1990). *The Indian Child Welfare Act: Indian Homes for Indian Children.* Los Angeles: UCLA American Indian Studies Center.

Kessel, J.A. & Robbins, S.P. (1984). The Indian Child Welfare Act: Dilemmas and needs. *Child Welfare, 63*(3), 225-232.

MacEachron, A.E. (1994). Supervision in tribal and state child welfare agencies: Professionalization, responsibilities, training needs, and satisfaction. *Child Welfare, 73*(2), 117-128.

MacEachron, A.E., Gustavsson, N.S., Cross, S., & Lewis, A. (1996). The effectiveness of the Indian Child Welfare Act of 1978. *Social Service Review, 70*(3), 451-463.

Mannes, M. (1995). Factors and events leading to the passage of the Indian Child Welfare Act. *Child Welfare, 74*(1), 264-282.

New York State Child Welfare Training Institute. (1992). *Culturally Competent Casework Practice.* Buffalo, NY: Center for Development of Human Services.

New York State Department of Social Services & State University of New York Research Foundation: Buffalo State College. (1996). Serving Children and Families through Native American Resources. Video and teleconference.

Public law 95-608. The Indian Child Welfare Act of 1978.

Steele, C.S. (1995). *Indian Child Welfare Act: An Instructional Guide for Judges and Judicial Educators.* Reno, NV: The National Judicial College.

U.S.C.A. 25, Chapter 21, Section 1901.

United States Senate Select Committee on Indian Affairs, Ninety-sixth Congress. (1980). *Oversight of the Indian Child Welfare Act.* Washington, D.C.: U.S. Government Printing Office.

United States House of Representatives Subcommittee on Indian Affairs and Public Lands, Ninety-fifth Congress. (1981). *Indian Child Welfare Act of 1978: To Establish Standards for the Placement of Indian Children in Foster or Adoptive Homes, to Prevent the Breakup of Indian Families, and for Other Purposes.* Washington, D.C.: U.S. Government Printing Office.

United States Senate Select Committee on Indian Affairs, Ninety-fifth Congress. (1977). *Indian Child Welfare Act of 1977: To Establish Standards for the Placement of Indian Children in Foster or Adoptive Homes, to Prevent the Breakup of Indian Families, and for Other Purposes.* Washington, D.C.: U.S. Government Printing Office.

United States Senate Select Committee on Indian Affairs, Ninety-eighth Congress. (1984). *Oversight of the Indian Child Welfare Act of 1978.* Washington, D.C.: U.S. Government Printing Office.

United States Senate Select Committee on Indian Affairs, One Hundredth Congress. (1988). *To Amend the Indian Child Welfare Act.* Washington, D.C.: U.S. Government Printing Office.

United States Senate Select Committee on Indian Affairs, One Hundred Fourth Congress. (1996). *Amendments to the Indian Child Welfare Act.* Washington, D.C.: U.S. Government Printing Office.

Wares, D.M., Dobrec, A., Rosenthal, J.A., & Wedel, K.R. (1992). Job satisfaction, practice skills, and supervisory skills of administrators of Indian Child Welfare programs. *Child Welfare, 71*(5), 405-418.

Wares, D.M., Wedel, K.R., Rosenthal, J.A., & Dobrec, A. (1994). Indian child welfare: A multicultural challenge. *Journal of Multicultural Social Work, 3*(3), 1-15.

Whose Genes Are They?
The Human Genome Diversity Project

Leota Lone Dog

SUMMARY. The Human Genome Diversity Project (HGDP) has targeted several hundred indigenous peoples worldwide as their source of genetic material. Proponents for this project claim that information derived by analyzing these materials may be used for a variety of purposes ranging from finding a cure for diabetes to resolving debates about human origins. However, the HGDP plan raises many issues for indigenous people. This paper describes the project as well as the possible ethical and policy implications for Native communities. *[Article copies available for a fee from The Haworth Document Delivery Service: 1-800-342-9678. E-mail address: getinfo@haworthpressinc.com]*

The Human Genome Diversity Project (HGDP) has targeted several hundred indigenous peoples worldwide as their source of genetic material. Proponents for the project claim that information derived from these materials will not only contribute to resolving debates about human evolution but aid in the advancement of medical science and technology. The urgency for implementing this project is predicated on the basis that these populations are in imminent danger of extinction. However, once their genetic material has been collected, their cell lines can be "immortalized" and stored in gene banks for continued evaluation. Discussions regarding the planning and implementation of the HGDP have yet to include members of these targeted indigenous populations. Nor have they provided a forum in which to

---

[Haworth co-indexing entry note]: "Whose Genes Are They? The Human Genome Diversity Project." Lone Dog, Leota. Co-published simultaneously in *Journal of Health & Social Policy* (The Haworth Press, Inc.) Vol. 10, No. 4, 1999, pp. 51-66; and: *Health and the American Indian* (ed: Priscilla A. Day and Hilary N. Weaver) The Haworth Press, Inc., 1999, pp. 51-66. Single or multiple copies of this article are available for a fee from The Haworth Document Delivery Service [1-800-342-9678, 9:00 a.m. - 5:00 p.m. (EST). E-mail address: getinfo@haworthpressinc.com].

© 1999 by The Haworth Press, Inc. All rights reserved.

discuss the long term implications genetic research and engineering will have on the future of these communities. The denial of equal access to information about or openly discussing the Project's aim creates an atmosphere of paternalism and raises the suspicion of indigenous peoples. While unopposed to scientific research, Native people have witnessed the negative ramifications that can result from scientific data because of its influence on public opinion and government policies.

THE HUMAN GENOME DIVERSITY PROJECT

Members of the project include a consortium of universities in North America and Europe, the U.S. National Institute of Health (N.I.H.) and an intergovernmental Human Genome Group. Project planners intend to "immortalize" blood samples that will be gleaned from indigenous populations in danger of extinction or disruption as integral genetic units. Targeted for the HGDP research are approximately 9000 ethnic communities which comprise 720 indigenous populations. They have been identified as close to extinction via acculturation, intermarriage, threatened with the influx of modern society or just literally dying out. It is for these reasons HGDP's researchers have declared an urgency for the project to proceed as quickly as possible. Collection of samples now, from "endangered" communities, will enable scientists to study them long after they disappear or before other societies infringe upon them and their uniqueness is lost.

In 1991 Dr. Allan Wilson and Dr. Luca Cavalli-Sforza conceived of a plan to survey the genetic diversity of humanity. The idea developed over 40 years ago when Cavalli-Sforza envisioned a project that would:

> ... study the genes of people among the world's varied ethnic groups and most isolated tribes. [He believes it will be possible] ... to trace humanity's history back to its origins–and construct the successive waves of human migration that have spread mankind throughout the globe. And in doing so, Cavalli-Sforza hoped to shed light on the way the genes of differing population groups control their susceptibility to killing diseases. (Perlman, p. A12)

By analyzing variances between people, globally, proponents for the project claim that the most important results will be in the studies of human disease. According to Mary-Claire King, a geneticist at the University of California at Berkeley:

> ... the project could study why genetically susceptible people develop certain diseases in some locales but not in others. One mystery, for example, is why Americans of African ancestry have a high risk of hypertension but native Africans do not. (Rensberger, p. A3)

However, despite these claims, the HGDP project raises several concerns for indigenous peoples. Who will have access to the project's data and samples and who will monitor how this information will be used? What will be the criteria for professional access to the data? As it stands now, indigenous communities will have no control over their genetic material once it is collected. In short, they will have no control over how their genes are used by others now or in the future.

Criteria for Inclusion and Methods for Collection

1. Groups should be aboriginal; which in the "New World" means those that were in place as of 1492.
2. Either language, geography, or endogamy (habit of marrying one's own tribe) will define a population.
3. Little recent interbreeding with other groups must be evident.
4. Local scientists, anthropologists or ethnologists, with expertise in that population's customs and mores, must be available before a population is considered.
5. Groups should be readily accessible so that samples can reach the laboratory within 48 hours. This rules out, for example, certain populations in Borneo that would take 2 to 3 weeks to reach a laboratory (Rural Advancement Foundation International [RAFI], March 1993, p. 3).

Collections of DNA samples from white blood cells, cheek scrapings and hair follicles will be extracted from approximately, but not limited to, 25 members selected from each population. All samples must reach a local laboratory within 48 hours. From there samples will be transferred to a storage facility in Europe or at the American Type

Culture Collection (ATCC) based in Rockville, Maryland (U.S.A.), the world's largest patent culture depository. In addition, samples will also be left with respective local national governments. The Rural Advancement Foundation International (RAFI) maintains that, with the estimated cost of $2,300 to collect each sample and the anticipated number of human specimens to be collected ranging between 10,000-15,000, the total cost of sample collection alone will be between $23 million and $35 million (RAFI, May 1993, p. 2). At present, it appears that the only funding the U.S. federal government has provided has been towards the HGDP Roundtable Discussions. However, "Cavalli-Sforza and his colleagues . . . hope to obtain more than $20 million from U.S. government agencies in the next five years to push their research" (*San Francisco Chronicle*, 4/21/93, p. A12).

Non-governmental funding has been obtained to establish a prototype for collection. Ms. Debra Harry reports that:

> The HGDP Project has secured a grant from the J.D. and C.T. MacArthur Foundation (despite the expressed opposition of Native leaders) in order to develop a model protocol for the collection of genetic samples from indigenous groups. (p. 15)

PROFIT POTENTIAL

HGDP is still more than a decade from completion but the race for capitalizing on the commercial prospects in the United States is underway. In fact, as reported in the *New York Times*, January 30, 1994, some members of the medical community, anticipating the creation of new medical techniques and drugs, based on this research, are entering into the medical marketplace and have raised millions of dollars by selling shares of stocks in their ventures. From the same article one geneticist proclaims, "This is like the wild West, where everyone was trying to stake a claim." In the last two years at least ten companies and organizations were founded and are pursuing technologies related to the Human Genome Project and HGDP including developing equipment and techniques for speeding up research and turning that knowledge into marketable drugs and therapies. Other countries have been slower to commercialize this research, therefore, some prominent overseas scientists, eager to reap a share in the profits, have allied themselves with American companies (Fisher, p. 18).

PATENTING OF HUMAN GENETIC MATERIAL

The U.S. patent law excludes the patenting of plants and animals other than micro-organisms, however, it does not exclude the patentability of their parts or alterations. Traditionally "products of nature" were not patentable, however, bioethicist Ned Hettinger explains:

> The product of nature doctrine has been rendered vacuous by allowing that the isolation, purification, or alteration of an entity or substance from its natural state which turns it into something not "found in nature." Thus genes are patentable when they are isolated from their "impure form" (mixed in with other DNA in an organism's cells). By placing foreign genes into organisms, these organisms also become "substantially altered" and hence patentable "works of man." Biotechnicians who newly alter, isolate, purify, modify, assist, and manipulate naturally occurring micro-organisms are thus eligible to apply for biopatents under U.S. and European laws. (RAFI, Jan/Feb 1994, p. 2)

Scientists use the term "human biological materials" to refer to replenishing substances (blood, skin, bone marrow, hair, urine, perspiration, semen, etc.) as well as non-replenishing parts (heart, kidney, etc.) in the body. The human materials most frequently used are tissues and cells. These "undeveloped" human materials are considered biological "inventions" and thus patentable once they are used to produce cell lines, hybridomas, and cloned genes.[1]

The precedent for the patenting of genetic material was set in 1980 when the U.S. Supreme Court rendered a landmark decision in the case of Diamond, Commissioner of Patents and Trademarks v. Chakrabarty.[2] Chakrabarty applied for a patent application for his invention of a human-made bacteria, which would be effective in controlling oil spills. The initial application was denied "on the grounds: (1) that micro-organisms are 'products of nature,' and (2) that as living things they are not patentable subject matter under 35 U.S.C. @101" (Diamond, p. 4). The Supreme Court's consideration of Title 35 U.S.C. @ 101 which provides for the issuance of a patent to a person who invents or discovers "any" new and useful "manufacture" or "composition of matter" ruled that the "respondent's micro-organism plainly qualifies as patentable subject matter. His claim is not to a hitherto unknown natural phenomena, but to a non-naturally occurring manufacture or composition of matter–a product of human ingenuity 'having a distinctive name [***13], character [and] [*310] use' " (Diamond, p. 7).[3]

Subsequent to this ruling, the patenting of micro-organisms has grown to include human genetic material.

- John Moore's "Mo Cell"

The 1979 case of John Moore reflects the ideology that now permeates the medical community. Patents for the "Mo" cell, as it has been coined, are held by the Sandoz pharmaceutical company and are valued at 1 billion dollars. The California Supreme Court denied that John Moore had rights to any profits of the potential pharmaceutical drugs derived from his cell line, ". . . which was found to produce high levels of useful (and profitable) proteins. . . . [The court inferred that] . . . he did *not* have rights of ownership over his cells after they had been removed from his body." (RAFI, Jan/Feb 1994, p. 7)

- The Al-Milano Gene

In the late 1970s researchers discovered what was termed the "Limone gene," which reduced the levels of HDL cholesterol in their blood plasma. They determined that approximately 30 members of the 1000 inhabitants of a small village in Limone, Italy were carriers of this mutant gene that appeared to protect them from heart disease. The mutation:

> is believed to have arisen spontaneously during the 18th century [and] was preserved through intermarriage between Limone residents. The village was separated from neighboring communities up until 1954 due to the lack of incoming roads. (Danheiser, p. 20)

Pharmaceutical companies in Europe became very interested in this discovery and saw the potential for the commercial development of medications to be used in combating cardiovascular disease, created from protein cloned from the gene. Patent applications have already been applied for by a Swedish pharmaceutical company which will allow them the exclusive rights for the production of drugs derived from the Limone gene.

In 1991, the National Institute of Health (NIH) applied for patents on more than 2,800 genes and DNA fragments in the human brain, despite the fact that the NIH scientists had no idea what function the gene sequences played in the human body. The potential knowledge and potential profits to be gained gave reason enough to try to establish exclusive rights.

The government and/or corporations conceivably stand to earn royalties from products derived from the genes of indigenous people who have been classified as endangered. Rather than pursuing efforts to save and protect these populations, they envision profits long after many of these communities have disappeared.

U.S. PATENT ON THE HUMAN CELL LINES OF INDIGENOUS PEOPLES

In August 1993, RAFI researchers found that the U.S. government had applied for a U.S. and world patent on the cell line of a 26-year-old Guaymi Indian woman from Panama (WO 9208784). In January 1994, they discovered that two more world patent claims were applied for by the U.S. government on indigenous people.[4]

In November 1993, the U.S. Secretary of Commerce, Ron Brown, withdrew the patent claim on the Guaymi woman's cell line. This was in response to international protest and action by the Guaymi General Congress and others. However, the cell line has not been returned and efforts are underway by the Panamanian government to call for its repatriation. Debra Harry reports that:

> The Solomon Islands Government has demanded withdrawal of the patent applications and repatriation of the genetic samples, citing an invasion of sovereignty, lack of informed consent, and moral grounds as the reasons for the protest. In early March, Secretary Ron Brown rejected these requests, stating that "there is no provision for considerations related to the source of the cells that may be the subject of a patent application." In other words, according to existing patent law, the source of a genetic sample is irrelevant. (p. 14)

Patent guidelines for subject matter have been redefined, as we have seen, "to include anything under the sun made by man," thus alterations of genetic materials are patentable. Additionally, once human genetic materials have been altered, they are no longer classified as "products of nature" and as in the case of John Moore are no longer the property of the source from which they were derived. The broadening of the definition of subject matter serves to deny ownership of a person's own genetic material, once it has been altered, as well as monetary compensation for how it is used.

Denying compensation to the communities who were the original source of these genetic materials is exploitation of the very fabric of our being and enters the realm of genetic imperialism. Furthermore, the long term ramifications of how our genetic samples may be used outside of the medical community could pose a potential threat for future generations. If this research is so important for humanity, the very least that should be offered is compensation or a guarantee of financial payment from any royalties to insure the physical, individual and actual survival of the "endangered" communities contributing to medical science.

While the advancement of genetic engineering will potentially introduce successful cures for many diseases, it conflicts with the religious and cultural values of Native Americans. Genetic manipulation of samples collected from indigenous peoples upsets the balance and the natural order of life. These beliefs as well as the reciprocal relationships with all creation are integral components of Native American spiritual and cultural systems. Furthermore, what threat to the environment does genetic engineering pose? Additionally, keeping in mind that we are all indigenous to the planet, what threat does this manipulation pose for everyone?

ETHICAL CONCERNS AND POLICY IMPLICATIONS

A new frontier is developing in the medical community at the expense of Indigenous people. Indigenous populations have been continually exploited in the name of progress. Now the possibility of enormous profits for both the scientific and business communities, through the colonization of indigenous genetic material without consideration for how indigenous people will benefit, is not acceptable.[5] In addition, collection methods that include bribery as well as the use of genetic material which would violate the spiritual beliefs of Native Americans are but two of the reasons to include our communities in establishing ethical and moral guidelines for this research.

Project planners have discussed the possibility of collecting samples from non-living persons as well as from fetal and placental tissue. They have stated:

> As to anonymous samples from dead people, the National Graves Protection and Repatriation Act in the United States provides rules for the return of skeletal remains. If you can identify an existing successor group to which the remains are related, that group's permission is necessary; if you cannot identify an existing group to which the remains are related, he [Dr. Kenneth Weiss, Professor of Anthropology at Pennsylvania State University] believes they may be used without permission. The use of fetal and placental tissue will, of course, be governed by local rules and morals. There is no blanket answer to whether you should be able to take samples from people who appear at isolated hospitals outside their homes. (HGDP, p. 6)

The NGPRA, however, is limited and as Cambria Ezell states, it:

> ... does not protect human remains located on state or privately owned lands and it does not affect the disposition of human remains or burial objects which are currently held by collectors who do not receive federal funds, or those items in any collection that were taken from state or privately owned lands. Therefore, in repatriation, policy makers weigh respect for the Native American's culture and religion against the scientific community's objectives of preservation, education, and research into past cultures through the use of remains as a source of material for health and native medicinal research. (Ezell, p. 13)

The colonization of Native genetic materials combined with scientific imperialism can render policies such as the NGPRA as symbolic rather than an act to fulfill the trust relationship and protection of Native American sovereignty. The disregard for important Native American policy sets dangerous precedents, reifying the racist ideologies embedded in scientific methodologies during the nineteenth century.

In the nineteenth century Samuel George Morton, one of America's leading craniologists, sought to test his hypothesis that racial ranking could be established objectively by the physical characteristics of the brain, particularly its size. Morton's collection of skulls was the largest in the world. Because of his interest in the Indigenous peoples in the Americas by the time of his death he had collected over 1,000 skulls. In 1939 he published the results of his data in a book titled *Crania Americana*. In it he not only included the data which confirmed his prior conviction of Caucasian superiority but also his conclusions on the inferior cultural characteristics of Native Americans. Stephen Jay Gould, author of *The Mismeasure of Man*, reanalyzed Morton's data and uncovered discrepancies. He found that the miscalculations of cranial medians as well as the unequal representation of the skulls selected for comparisons allowed Morton to formulate the conclusions that would support his prior convictions. Gould found no evidence of fraud; however, he states that:

> The prevalence of *unconscience finagling* . . . suggests a general conclusion about the social context of science. For if scientists can be honestly self-deluded to Morton's extent, then prior prejudice may be found anywhere, even in the basics of measuring bones and toting sums. (Gould, pp. 55-56)

Misuse of genetic information can serve to support racist and nationalistic claims and, in effect, facilitate the institutionalization of such claims for setting national policy. As an example, a study performed in Europe between 1900 and 1950, which evaluated the geographical distribution of blood groups, produced the Hizfeld Index. This index evaluated a population's percentage of type A blood divided by its percentage of type B blood. The highest percentage of type A blood was found in northern and western Europe. The Hizfeld study demonstrated a high incidence of the type A blood group in northern Europe and of the type B blood group in southern Europe. This study was used by "Aryans" in Germany and other groups in the 1930s to justify a population hierarchy and to establish Germany as the nation which was blocking the invasion of, what they judged to be, inferior type B blooded individuals from the east and south of Europe (HGDP, p. 20). Genetic discrimination could be the future criteria for establishing racist policy.

The knowledge of and access to an indigenous community's unique genetic make-up makes it theoretically possible to devise biological weapons to wage genetic warfare against specific human communities. Governments will have access, as well, and could very well use this information to control or further endanger the survival of indigenous populations within their borders. Biological warfare has been effective in the past against indigenous people in the United States and was used during the French and Indian War. Sharon O'Brien relates:

> In a last ditch attempt to contain the British, the great Ottawa leader Pontiac inspired eighteen tribes from western Pennsylvania and northern Ohio into a powerful alliance. In well-planned, spontaneous attacks in 1763, Pontiac and his warriors captured eight of the ten British forts east of Fort Niagara. Two thousand British troops and settlers were killed in the attack. Sir Jeffrey Amherst, commander in chief of the British forces in North America, in perhaps the first example of biological warfare, retaliated by sending "gifts" of small-pox infected blankets to the tribes allied with the French. (pp. 46-47)

Similar tactics were used to gain possession of the land from Native people. In many instances, unscrupulous politicians used alcohol as a means to manipulate particular situations. For example:

> William Henry Harrison, governor of Indiana from 1801 to 1811 (and later president) bribed a few unauthorized chiefs with alcohol and negotiated a treaty that ceded three million acres of land, including land from tribes not even represented at the council. (O'Brien, p. 53)

Now, comparable tactics are being considered by HGDP researchers to appropriate indigenous genetic samples. For many indigenous communities who are struggling to survive, the offer of life-sustaining necessities would be an incentive that might compromise the willingness of community members to participate. Monetary compensation would appear to be the most coercive "reward," however, in many communities Cavalli-Sforza found:

> In his recent genetic studies of Pygmies, . . . the villagers were extremely reluctant to let him take blood samples because they feared they would be giving him power over them. But when he brought them modern medicines they needed, the villagers were willing participants in his research. As a result, Cavalli-Sforza believes that in return for the willing participation of the people his project will study, he and his colleagues must be prepared to offer modern medical care. (Perlman, p. A12)

Cavalli-Sforza does not appear to be aware of the morally corrupt precedent being set by this means of obtaining participation. The quest for scientific research has begun to supersede the value of human life. Researchers heralding the future benefits to be derived from indigenous genetic samples is of little benefit to people who are suffering now. Limited access to affordable modern medical care is one of the direct causes that challenges their quality of life and the ability to survive. One must ask, will the funds used to support HGDP's research and laboratories be redirected from other essential projects that would support and sustain indigenous communities?

CONCLUSION

HGDP researchers assert that the study of indigenous genetic material will contribute to the advancement of mankind. However, will indigenous communities be able to reap the benefits of medical research resulting from their genetic material? If these communities are alive, will they be able to afford the advanced medical technology that would not have existed without them? The veil of secrecy surrounding the HGDP raises suspicions for many indigenous peoples and exclusion from the discussion and planning process compounds our suspicions about the real motives fueling this research and raises the question about their willingness to operate on an ethical and moral level. In addition, we must consider the possibility of legislative action which could present the conflict of maintaining one's ethics while operating within the domain of the law, which may be unethical. Enslavement was legal in this country, but unethical. It was also legal to forcibly remove entire nations of Indian people, confine them to reservations and enact policies to forcibly eradicate their culture, but this too was unethical. What is in store for indigenous populations? What theories will this research engender? There are many questions which must be addressed before our communities can even consider the possibility of cooperating with this project.

The possibility of an open access policy means scientists will only have to demonstrate the validity of their research in requesting samples. How will the data derived from these studies be used? As in the case of Morton, how can we possibly scrutinize the intentions of scientists conducting their research? Will new research be used to create new stereotypes or further existing ones? How will data derived from genetic research be reflected in future sociopolitical ideology? Will ethics be compromised in order to achieve scientific ends and/or legalize sociopolitical policies? What will be the impact of new evolutionary migratory claims? How will they affect the land claims of indigenous peoples in North America? As a result of HGDP research, will tribal recognition and identification policies be predicated on DNA samples? Will new discriminatory practices towards indigenous peoples be developed based on the discovery of genetically based diseases? Or, conversely, will the discovery of genetically based solutions to current diseases engender the appropriation of indigenous genetic material?

Thus, the policy implications of this research for Native Americans are profound. Acts such as the NGPRA or policies regarding land claims, and ultimately tribal self-determination, could be undermined by precedents set forth in the HGDP plan. What appears to be an innocuous proposal to further science is in reality a dangerous proposal which can set a precedent to undermine Native American policies that protect tribal sovereignty and self-determination.

Research predicated on the assumption that *they* and not we know what is best for our communities as well as a reluctance to be forthright reinforces the continuation of paternalistic and colonizing attitudes towards indigenous communities. Therefore, despite the low level publicity surrounding the Human Genome Diversity Project, indigenous people in North America are becoming increasingly aware that, regardless of its goals, it is not advisable that we participate until we have more information. Even with additional information it is our right to determine whether our communities will participate. For today it is not our bones that are being collected for examination but our genes!

NOTES

1. The following terms, as defined by RAFI, are three of the most common "inventions" based on human genetic material:
   • Human Cell Line:
   A sample of cells removed from the human body that are capable of sustaining continuous, long term growth in cultures. Cell lines are said to be "immortal" because they can continue to live indefinitely under artificial conditions (with strict control of temperature, nutrient requirements, and sterile conditions). Human cell lines provide an inexhaustible supply of DNA (the complete genetic code) of the individual from whom they are taken.

- Cloned Genes:
Using genetic engineering, scientists can isolate a human gene or fragment of human DNA and make many copies of it by inserting it into cells (which can be from a non-human species) and letting it multiply. Cloned material can be used to examine how a biological process is regulated, identify and isolate scarce compounds, or produce commercial quantities of important substances. Many patents are being granted for DNA sequences coding for the production of human proteins for biomedicine. Examples of genetically engineered products created through gene cloning are: human growth hormone, human insulin, and human alpha interferon.
- Hybridomas:
A hybrid cell that is capable of multiplying continuously in culture and supplying a specific type of antibody. The hybridoma cell results from the fusion of a particular type of immortal tumor cell line (a myeloma) with an antibody-producing white blood cell (B lymphocyte). The antibodies secreted by hybridomas, known as monoclonal antibodies, have revolutionized the way that human illnesses are diagnosed and treated (RAFI, Jan/Feb. 1994, p. 3).

2. In 1971, General Electric and one of its employees, Ananda Mohan Chakrabarty, applied for the U.S. patent on a genetically engineered Pseudomonas bacteria. Taking plasmids from three kinds of bacteria he transplanted them into a fourth. As he explained, "I simply shuffled genes, changing bacteria that already existed." The patent office rejected the application on the basis that animate life forms were not patentable. The case was appealed in the Court of Customs and Patent Appeals Office and the Supreme Court nine years later. Chakrabarty was granted his patent on the grounds that the microorganism was not a product of nature, but Chakrabarty's invention and therefore patentable. As Andrew Kimble, a leading U.S. lawyer, recounts, "In coming to its precedent-shattering decision, the court seemed unaware that the inventor himself had characterized his 'creation' of the microbe as simply 'shifting' genes, not creating life" (Shiva, pp. 2-3).

3. ". . . this Court has read the term 'manufacture' in @101 in accordance with its dictionary definition to mean 'the production of articles for use from raw or prepared materials by giving to these materials new forms, qualities, properties, or combinations, whether by hand-labor or by machinery' ." . . . Similarly, "composition of matter" has been construed consistent with its common usage to include "all compositions of two or more substances and . . . all composite articles, whether they be the results of chemical union, or of mechanical mixture, or whether they be gases, fluids, powders or solids." . . . In choosing such expansive terms as "manufacture" and "composition of matter," modified by the comprehensive "any," Congress plainly contemplated that the patent laws would be given wide scope. . . . The Patent Act of 1793, authored by Thomas Jefferson, defined [***11] statutory subject matter as "any new and useful art, machine, manufacture, or composition of matter, or any new or useful improvement [thereof]." . . . . In 1952, when the patent laws were recodified . . . Congress intended statutory subject matter [**2208] to "include anything under the sun made by man" (Diamond, p. 6).

4. RAFI reports that:
The first patent application (Publication Number WO93/03759), filed in the

name of the US Department of Health and Human Services and the National Institutes of Health, stakes claim to the human T-cell line of a Papua New Guinean. According to the patent application, blood samples were taken from 24 people who belong to the Hagahai people of Madang Province, New Guinea, in May, 1989. The cell line, the first of its kind from an individual from Papua New Guinea, is potentially useful in treating or diagnosing individuals infected with an HTLYV-1 variant virus. 24 Human T-lymphotropic virus type 1 (HTLY-1) is associated with adult leukemia and with a chronic degenerative neurologic disease. The novel cell line is of potential value in understanding the enhancement or suppression of an immune response to this virus. The second patent claim (WO-9215325-A), filed in the name of the US Department of Commerce, is for the human T-cell line of a 40-year-old woman from the Marovo Lagoon in Western Province and a 58-year-old man from Guadalcanal Province, both of the Solomon Islands. Blood samples were taken in March and August 1990. Similar to the patent claim mentioned above, the cell line may be useful in producing vaccines and/or diagnosing human T-lymphotropic virus type 1. The human cell lines derived from blood samples taken from Papua New Guineans and the Solomon Islanders are now on deposit at the ATCC (RAFI, Jan/Feb 1994, pp. 7-8).

5. These concerns were expressed in the Final Report of the Haudenosaunee and Teton Sioux Nation Treaty Council Delegations on the XIth Session–Working Group on Indigenous Populations. July 19-31, 1993, Geneva, Switzerland.

REFERENCES

Danheiser, Susan L. (1993, January 15). Low Levels of Mutant HDLs in Italian Town Appear to Ward Off Cardiovascular Disease. *Genetic Engineering News, 13* (2), 1, 20.
Diamond, Commissioner of Patents and Trademarks v. Chakrabarty, No. 79-136. (1994). Lexis-Nexis. Services of Mead Data Central, Inc.
Ezell, Cambria. (1994, August). Human Genome Diversity Project and Native American Religious and Privacy Rights. *American Indian Law Alliance,* p. 13.
Fisher, Lawrence A. (1994, January 30). Profits and Ethics Clash in Research on Genetic Coding. *The New York Times, Late Edition,* pp. 1, 18.
Gould, Stephen Jay. (1981). *The Mismeasure of Man.* New York: W.W. Norton & Company.
Harry, Debra. (1995). The Human Genome Diversity Project: Implications for Indigenous Peoples. *Perspectives on Biodiversity and Intellectual Property, 8* (4), pp. 13-15.
Human Genome Diversity Project: Summary of Planning Workshop 3(B): Ethical and Human Rights Implications. (1993, February 16-18). Transcript, pp. 20-30. U.S. National Institutes of Health in Bethesda, Maryland.
Morton, Samuel George. (1839). *Crania Americana: or A Comparative View of the Skulls of Various Aboriginal Nations of North and South America. To Which Is Prefixed an Essay of the Varieties of the Human Species.* Philadelphia.

O'Brien, Sharon. (1989). *American Indian Tribal Governments.* Norman: Oklahoma UP.
Perlman, David. (1993, April 21). Genetic Sleuths Race Against Time. *San Francisco Chronicle*, pp. A1, 12.
RAFI Communique. (1993, March). The Vampire Documentation. Reference: franthro.wp/B47 9, pp. 1-7.
RAFI Communique. (1993, May). Patents, Indigenous Peoples, and Human Genetic Diversity. pp. 1-6.
RAFI Communique. (1993, October 25). Indigenous People Protest U.S. Secretary of Commerce Patent Claim on Guaymi Indian Cell Line. pp. 1-2.
RAFI Communique. (1994, January/February). The Patenting of Human Genetic Material. pp. 1-12.
Rensberger, Boyce. (1993, February 22). Science: Molecular Anthropology Tracking the Parade of Mankind via Clues in the Genetic Code. *The Washington Post, Final Edition*, p. A03.
Shiva, Vandana. (1993, December). Patenting of Life Forms: Why Ecologists Should Worry About the Dunkel Draft. *Ecology*, pp. 2-3.

Interactions Between American Indian Ethnicity and Health Care

Wynne DuBray, PhD
Adelle Sanders, MSW

SUMMARY. Interventions in health care must be sensitive to the part that culture plays in treatment, recovery and healing of the American Indian patient. Cultural factors play an important part in how the family participates and copes with the intervention program. Interpreting communication and behavior from the perspective of the family's culture contributes to positive family-professional interaction.

This paper addresses the most important cultural factors impinging on positive health care for American Indian families and addresses a process for assessment of cultural conflicts which may prevent positive outcomes in the delivery of health care to this population. In addition, this paper offers strategies throughout that can be used by health care professionals to assure culturally sensitive service delivery to American Indians. *[Article copies available for a fee from The Haworth Document Delivery Service: 1-800-342-9678. E-mail address: getinfo@haworthpressinc.com]*

Intervention in health care must be sensitive to cultural nuances which may influence the interactions between provider and client. Culture and ethnicity are tightly interwoven. Culture is broadly defined as a set of possibilities from which the family may choose (Anderson & Fenichel, 1989). More specifically, culture refers to all that people have learned to do, to value, and to enjoy from their history, hence it is the shared patterns of learned behavior, both implicit and explicit, or the transmitted symbols representing the achieve-

---

[Haworth co-indexing entry note]: "Interactions Between American Indian Ethnicity and Health Care." DuBray, Wynne and Adelle Sanders. Co-published simultaneously in *Journal of Health & Social Policy* (The Haworth Press, Inc.) Vol. 10, No. 4, 1999, pp. 67-84; and: *Health and the American Indian* (ed: Priscilla A. Day and Hilary N. Weaver) The Haworth Press, Inc., 1999, pp. 67-84. Single or multiple copies of this article are available for a fee from The Haworth Document Delivery Service [1-800-342-9678, 9:00 a.m. - 5:00 p.m. (EST). E-mail address: getinfo@haworthpressinc.com].

© 1999 by The Haworth Press, Inc. All rights reserved.

ments of a particular historical group; therefore, it becomes the framework that guides all life practices (Crowe, 1997). Ethnicity, on the other hand, is the social or cultural heritage shared by a particular group, which relates to the group's customs, language, religion, and habits that are passed on from generation to generation (Crowe, 1997). However, a family's cultural identity does not always dictate how the family will respond to a health crisis. Many combined factors are involved. Professionals must therefore be careful to avoid stereotyping clients of color and making assumptions that all members of a particular cultural group will react in a predetermined manner.

Any generalizations made about different cultural groups, such as American Indians, are only valid when they are considered in the broadest sense of the term. The effective health care provider acknowledges the importance of culture and ethnicity, learns the general characteristics of those cultures, and realizes that cultural factors will play an important part in how the family participates in and copes with the intervention program.

The most important contribution that cultural knowledge adds to the equation is to help the professional be aware of cultural differences and cultural conflicts. Practices that may seem odd to the professional are often seen as logical within the context of the family's culture, since disability, health, and wellness are assigned different definitions within the context of culture (Crowe, 1997). Therefore, interpreting communication and behavior from the perspective of the family's culture contributes to a more positive family-professional interaction. Effective interventions are based upon respect for the family's culture. Families should be given the opportunity to take the lead in expressing how their culture is executed within their family.

DEGREE OF ACCULTURATION

Acculturation is a form of adaptation whereby members of an ethnic cultural group relinquish some, if not all, of the elements of their cultural identity and become immersed into the dominant society's culture (Locke, 1992; Lum, 1996). People of various ethnic groups achieve varying degrees of acculturation in order to survive in the dominant society. The health care practitioner needs to be aware that acculturation has an impact on how the family views the health care issues confronting it, as well as the relationship between the family and the health care practitioner. There exist several levels of acculturation (Locke, 1992; Lum, 1996). For the purpose of this paper, these levels of acculturation may be reframed into three main categories of acculturation, which best describe the effects of acculturation on American Indians:

Traditional: In the traditional form of acculturation, the traditional language and customs of the root culture are strongly maintained in spite of exposure to the dominant culture. These individuals or families, often but not necessarily, continue to live in non-urban settings, and their psychological, social, political, and economic needs are met almost exclusively within their ethnic community.

Assimilated: In the assimilated form of acculturation, individuals or families have acquired and emulate the behavioral patterns, lifestyles, values, and language of the dominant culture. Generally, they seek to meet their needs outside of their ethnic culture. Socio-economic and educational factors have often, but not always, played a significant part in this movement away from the ethnic culture and into the culture of power, the dominant society. As a result of this acculturation, many assimilated American Indians do not identify themselves as "American Indian."

Bicultural: In this form of acculturation, individuals and families have acquired traits of the dominant group, but they also retain many of the ethnic characteristics, values, and beliefs of their tribal group, therefore, they are equally comfortable in both worlds and live and socialize in integrated settings. These individuals and families have a dual commitment, a loyalty to their communities of origin and a stake in the political and economic institutions of the dominant society. By and large, they are able to move fluidly and comfortably from one language and/or culture to the other.

This paper will address the needs of American Indian clients who fall into the Traditional and Bicultural groups. The Assimilated American Indians are usually comfortable with mainstream services provided to Anglo clients, since they usually do not identify with the American Indian community or culture. To provide adequate levels of services to American Indians, it is necessary for the health care provider to first assess the level of acculturation of the client being served in order to provide culturally sensitive services, and to do this, it is first necessary to gain knowledge about the effects of acculturation on American Indians, as well as an understanding of the history and cultural nuances of the tribal cultures.

AMERICAN INDIAN DEMOGRAPHICS

To gain this preliminary knowledge, one must begin with an understanding about who comprises the American Indian population within the United States. The designator "American Indians" in this paper refers to all North American native people, including Alaskan Natives, Aleuts, Eskimos, and mixed bloods. The American Indian population, which once was estimated at ten to fifteen million at the time of initial Anglo contact, diminished to approximately two million (DuBray, 1993). Approximately 400,000 Indian people (or 20%) are under the age of 15 (United States Department of Commerce, Bureau of Census, 1990). In addition, 39% of the American Indian population is under the age of 20, and the mean age among the American Indian population is 26 years, which is considerably younger than the United States median age of 33 years (United States Department of Commerce, Bureau of Census, 1990). American Indians have seen dramatic increases in population in recent years, with a 72% increase between 1970 and 1980 and another 38% increase between 1980 and 1990 (United States Department of Commerce, Bureau of Census, 1990). American Indians are thus considered one of the fastest growing populations today (Locke, 1992). In addition, there are 517 federally recognized native tribes in the United States, and each of these tribes maintains unique customs, traditions, and social organizations (LaFromboise, 1988). Furthermore, there are 200 distinct tribal languages currently spoken (Leap, 1981).

Due to economic factors and forced assimilation policies that have historically impacted this group, more than half of all American Indians live in urban areas today (United States Department of Commerce, Bureau of Census, 1990). This increased movement to urban areas has complicated the functioning of Indian extended family systems, resulting in many urban Indians feeling isolated from their extended families, and consequently, they have formed intertribal networks in the cities, which replicate this missing family system (DuBray, 1992).

THE AMERICAN INDIAN FAMILY AS MEDIATOR OF CULTURE

They were a people beginning with beliefs,
Ornament, language, fables, love of children
And a scheme of life that worked.

-Stephen Vincent Benet (1943)

Although American Indians vary widely in tribal traditions and languages, they have many common values and characteristics. Additionally, they share a history of oppression, genocide, and discrimination as "conquered" aboriginal Americans. Spirituality is the common thread that links together the many aspects of a philosophy of life that worked for thousands of years before contact with the invaders. The powers of nature, the personal quest of the soul, the solidarity of the tribe, the acts of cooperation in daily life all are spiritual, and all are sustained by dance and ritual (DuBray, 1992, 1993; Steer, 1996; Allen, 1991).

Although American Indians are at different levels of acculturation, as aforementioned, there still remains a strong desire among the Traditional and Bicultural American Indians to be with their own people and to preserve their inner values and cultural integrity. It is because of this desire for maintaining their cultural identity and connectedness to each other that American Indians owe their record of survival throughout the many centuries of encroachment upon their lives and land by a more numerous and a more aggressive race (Debo, 1970). However, this constant battle to maintain their homelands and to preserve their cultural identity has taken its toll upon American Indian families. Declining health and stress related illnesses are prevalent in most tribal communities (DuBray, 1992, 1993). Poorly funded educational institutions and substandard health facilities contribute to high rates of unemployment, poverty, and poor health for the majority of American Indians living on reservations today (DuBray, 1992, 1993).

Despite pressures from missionary boarding schools to assimilate American Indian children, and federal governmental policies enacted to force assimilation upon Indian people, American Indians have resisted this effort to melt them into the dominant American society in most of their communities (DuBray, 1993). In addition, the family unit has remained the chief conveyor of culture for several hundred years, and this family unit includes grandparents, aunts, uncles, cousins, and sometimes adopted relatives. Parenting is shared, resources are shared, social control is strong, and elders hold prominent positions in families. This sustaining influence of the American Indian family over transmitting culture must be recognized as a strength by health care practitioners, when working with American Indian families. Not utilizing this strength to work with families in this community will result in resistance from the American Indian client family to the health care intervention (Clark, Zales & Sacco, 1982; Anderson & Stewart, 1983).

As the primary agent of socialization and the conveyor of culture, the American Indian family prepares the child for adult responsibilities at an early age. American Indian children are taught to prepare meals, to complete household chores, to care for the sick and elderly, and to follow in their parents' footsteps. Furthermore, children are taught to respect their elders, and they are praised for good behavior, rather than punished for wrong behavior (Locke, 1992; DuBray, 1992, 1993). Appropriate behavior and family manners are usually modeled by parents without extensive verbal communication explaining the preferred behavior (Locke, 1992; DuBray, 1992, 1993). Disapproval can be sensed by the child through non-verbal signals from the parents or elders when unacceptable behavior is demonstrated. This non-verbal communication is not usually noticed or understood by people outside of the culture, who are more focused on verbal communication and its content rather than the process. It would be important for health professionals to become more aware of these non-verbal communication patterns in order to correctly read messages being sent and received through these channels of communication, which could have an impact on the health care intervention being implemented (Crowe, 1997). Learning to listen to what American Indians are saying through body language can teach the health care practitioner much about acceptance of, or resistance to, the proposed intervention (Sue & Sue, 1990).

CULTURE SHAPES BELIEFS AND BEHAVIORAL PATTERNS IN TRADITIONAL AND BICULTURAL FAMILIES

Variations in beliefs and behaviors are found both within and between cultural groups, including among American Indians (Locke, 1992). An American Indian family may find the extended family a source of support and identity, and therefore, in many tribal cultures, the elders and grandparents have significant control over adult children and the raising of grandchildren (Ashford et al., 1997). Because of the historical antecedents of removal and extermination of American Indians by the federal government, as well as the many forced assimilation policies imposed upon this group by the government, American Indians are slow to trust Euro-American health professionals (Green, 1982). Consequently, it is necessary for health care professionals to learn about the family's language and tribal cultural customs by first reading existing literature, and then conferring with members of the tribal community about their culture, thereby developing an understanding of the different beliefs and attitudes before working with the American Indian patient (Crowe, 1997).

Because behavior is learned through modeling, child rearing practices are passed on from one generation to the next (Locke, 1992). Communication patterns of American Indian tribal groups have many common characteristics as a result of this intergenerational transfer of knowledge. Consequently, among tribal people, language is usually spoken softly and briefly, and much communication is indirect with little questioning or probing for additional information. Long pauses in conversation are common as Indian people have learned to be comfortable with silence (DuBray, 1992, 1993). Furthermore, many Indian clients will withdraw when there is disagreement in relationships with dominant society health care professionals, rather than argue their point. This learned passive behavioral expression is the result of not experiencing positions of power and control in relationships within the dominant society and being severely sanctioned for expressing themselves during their long history of survival. In addition, cooperation is a strong value as opposed to competition, which means that if the situation is confrontational or threatening, American Indians will not participate in it (DuBray, 1992, 1993). If the health care professional becomes knowledgeable in the area of cultural styles of expression, mis-communications will be avoided, thereby promoting a positive family-professional relationship, which will result in improved health care delivery (Crowe, 1997).

Each tribal group has traditions and customs pertaining to family roles, child rearing, marriage, spiritual ceremonies, rites of passage, family responsibilities, and grieving for the deceased (DuBray, 1993). Spiritual ceremonies are closely connected to the healing of the sick in many tribal cultures (DuBray, 1993; Lum, 1996). This may involve purification ceremonies such as the "Sweat Lodge" or other healing ceremonies performed to heal specific illnesses (DuBray, 1993). It would be important for health care professionals to explore the importance of these culturally ingrained spiritual practices with their clients. Becoming aware of the alternative health care practices being used assists the health care practitioner in fully addressing the health care needs of the American Indian client (DuBray, 1993; Crowe, 1997).

All tribes believe in the intrinsic worth of the individual. Such conditions as Fetal Alcohol Syndrome and its resulting mental retardation do not lead to rejection of American Indian children by their families. The child is valued to the same degree as other children in the family and tribe (Anderson & Fenichel, 1989; Garrison & McQuiston, 1989; Hendren & Berlin, 1991; Sullivan, 1983). This is a departure from cultures where the intellect of children and college educations are seen as necessary for acceptance by their families. Likewise, children born with other physical defects are not seen as less than acceptable by their families, nor are the mentally ill ostracized, which often happens in families of other cultures (DuBray, 1993). This knowledge would assist the health care practitioner in understanding an American Indian's perception about what is illness, as well as understanding the resistance to standard medical labels that the health care profession assigns.

Indian people value the group over the individual (DuBray, 1992). Therefore, when decisions are made, the family is consulted, and the family has much more influence over these decisions being made about an individual family member needing health care than one sees in Euro-American cultures. The idea of being a "rugged individual" is not held as a value within most tribes. The separation/individuation process described in Euro-American psychological literature does not pertain to the American Indian culture. In fact, in many Indian tribes, the adolescent and young adult offspring remain in the family home to form their own household, and the young adult remains obedient to the dictates of the family elders (Ashford et al., 1997).

Most tribal people believe it is important to live in harmony with nature and the environment. This means having respect for the earth, animals, trees, rocks, and all other living "things." Many unacculturated tribal groups value a present time orientation, which involves enjoying the "now" and experiencing whatever is happening in the present, rather than being preoccupied with either the past or the future (DuBray, 1992). Time is always with us, and people are more important to visit with than rushing off to be at a particular place at a specific time. In addition, the group as a whole decides when meetings are to start and when they are to be adjourned (DuBray, 1992).

This different time frame is in direct opposition to the Euro-American convention of linear time and can become a real bone of contention if it is not understood. Families may drop in for appointments, come on a different day, or come at a later time than scheduled. These behaviors are not deliberate acts performed to irritate staff, but they are common behavioral characteristics of tribal culture, and these behavioral characteristics are more likely to be manifested among the Traditional Acculturated American Indian subgroup than among the Bicultural Acculturated American Indian subgroup. The effective health care professional will understand that these families' attitudes toward time, spiritual harmony, and life forces are deeply embedded in the culture and have become a part of their lifestyle. Unfortunately, health institutions usually conform to Euro-American ways of living and doing business and have become, for the most part, directive and rigid. It might be useful, if health care professionals have a large number of Traditional American Indians on their caseloads, to consider alternative scheduling practices, or if there are only a few Traditional American Indians on the caseload, accommodating these clients within the context of the health care practice might be the solution to the problem of providing effective health care to this population.

Many American Indians embrace a "being" philosophy of life rather than that of "doing" (DuBray, 1992). The "doing" philosophy of life places demands on individuals to accomplish tasks based upon measurable standards perceived to be external to the acting individual. The "being" philosophy of life demonstrates a preference for spontaneous expression of what is recognized as a "given" in the human personality, a non-developmental conception. This helps explain why

American Indian parents do not pressure their children to achieve, but allow the children to move at their individual pace and to select their preferred life work based upon their own idea about what they want in life. Most American Indians are not impressed by college degrees or wealth. The "being" philosophy of life is in harmony with spirituality, non-materialistic lifestyles, and the intrinsic worth of the individual (DuBray, 1992). The "being" philosophy of life is also in harmony with a present time orientation, as well as in harmony with a nature orientation (DuBray, 1992). These are very important cultural attitudes and values that often are not understood by dominant culture health care professionals. To promote better communication, to foster positive regard for the American Indian, and to improve health care delivery, it would behoove health care providers to become culturally aware of these differences.

AMERICAN INDIAN SPIRITUALITY AND HEALING PERSPECTIVE

In reviewing the cultural values of the American Indian population and the importance of spirituality across all tribes, a modality which incorporates mind, body, and spirit is important (DuBray, 1992, 1993). This holistic perspective alleviates the sense of fragmentation which permeates American society today.

American Indian value systems dictate a model of growth and health which is useful for viewing the delivery of health care services, whether the target of the services is preventative, treating common health care conditions, or addressing chronic illness. The biological elements are viewed as less important than the historical and spiritual elements of humanity (Ashford et al., 1997). Therefore, the reductive and analytical view of humanity is replaced by one which synthesizes spiritual content and recognizes the purposive nature of humanity (DuBray, 1993; Ashford et al., 1997).

Since many American Indians believe in visions, rely on dreams for guidance from the spirits, and experience what is considered paranormal phenomena on a regular basis, a different reality evolves (DuBray, 1992). This reality has at its foundation a variety of old spiritual values and beliefs (DuBray, 1992). The elders are the keepers of the traditions and the guides to traditional culture (Steer, 1996). Consequently, Indian spirituality can be very different from the Christian belief systems. Many Indian people rely on medicine men and women for spiritual guidance. These spiritual counselors provide the American Indian client with a "Second Opinion," a most significant point of which health care professionals should be aware. In most tribes, spiritual leaders are male, although in many tribes, such as the Cherokee, these spiritual leaders can be elderly, post-menopausal women (Allen, 1991; Speer, 1996). In many of the California tribes, some women are the shamans (Allen, 1991; Lake, 1991). The causes of illness are sometimes attributed to an imbalance in one's body, mind, or spirit (Topper, 1987). To recreate health in the American Indian experiencing illness and adhering to these traditional beliefs, the health care professional must address the person in the context of the "whole," the body, mind, and spirit. This sometimes means that the health care professional must form a partnership with spiritual healers to affect the change in the health of the client; but, at least minimally, the health care professional must respect the spiritual practice being sought by the traditional Indian through the use of these spiritual healers.

NATURAL HEALING LEVELS

Many American Indians believe that individuals have within their constitution a natural healing system which can be mediated internally or externally (DuBray, 1993). A tribal ceremony can be a catalyst, setting in motion this healing process (DuBray, 1992, 1993). An example of a healing ceremony is the Sun Dance ceremony of the Lakota, which is conducted yearly to promote renewal and healing for an entire community (Lake, 1991). Many individuals have experienced healing of both physical and emotional ailments during this ceremony. Most American Indians are hesitant to discuss these healing ceremonies, as they are considered sacred by the tribe and, also, because the dominant society has long devalued such ceremonies and even imposed severe sanctions against Indians who practiced them. Another example of the impact these sacred practices can have on individuals involves an American Indian adolescent who was experiencing disturbing psychotic symptoms, but refused to take his prescribed medication, even at the urging of his parents. However, after a meeting with his medicine man, who prescribed tossing sacred corn toward the rising sun each morning, the young man was willing to take his medication because it was not replacing his religious belief (Hendren &

Berlin, 1991). Furthermore, many American Indians carry medicine pouches with them for spiritual reasons. These items should not be taken from them because to do so would be considered an infringement upon their religious freedom and could, in fact, cause greater illness and even death. Health professionals should support and validate tribal ceremonies as important to the American Indian family and should respect them as contributing to resiliency from crisis. By doing this, health care professionals will promote wellness in the holistic sense and will facilitate healing within a traditional context, which will promote positive interactions between the Indian client and the health care practitioner.

In addition to traditional spiritual practices, it is also important for health care professionals to be aware that many American Indians attended missionary schools and have integrated the Christian religion within their tribal customs. Therefore, because they identify as Christian does not mean that they do not also adhere to traditional practices, hence the client should have freedom to express both the traditional and/or the Christian perspectives within the context of healing. American Indians place great importance on spirituality, whether practiced through traditional ceremonies and/or through Christianity, and the importance of this spirituality is essential for health care professionals to bear in mind when treating clients from the American Indian community.

CONTRIBUTIONS OF THE EXTENDED FAMILY IN PROMOTING RESILIENCE

To provide valuable health care services to American Indians, it is important for health care professionals to become knowledgeable about the American Indian family and its parenting roles and practices, because the family plays an instrumental part in health care delivery, particularly with regard to the acceptance or rejection of the recommended interventions. In many American Indian families, grandparents, uncles, aunts, and cousins play a supportive role at times of crisis, especially illness. As aforementioned, grandparents may play an important role in the treatment planning for their grandchildren. They usually have great influence over their adult children and serve as counselors and natural helpers to others in the community (DuBray, 1992, 1993; Ashford et al., 1997). Furthermore, since most tribes originally lived in communal settings, the residuals of sharing resources are still prevalent in most tribes (DuBray, 1992). Generosity is a value, whether it involves giving of one's time or finances (DuBray, 1992). In addition, American Indians have strong family ties, which translates into family responsibilities for providing emotional and financial support to family members suffering from illness, chronic or otherwise. The extended family is very powerful in guiding and protecting its members in the American Indian community (Ashford et al., 1997). The extended family gives the American Indian client a sense of belonging and protection, and it serves as a symbolic blanket of emotional and spiritual security. Being clear on the importance of the extended family to the American Indian will facilitate health care professionals in providing quality health care services to Indian patients. Involving the extended family in planning the treatment intervention and its implementation will increase the likelihood of a successful health outcome (Anderson & Stewart, 1988; Green, 1982; Sullivan, 1983; Paterson, 1982).

THE FAMILY SYSTEMS APPROACH TO INTERVENTION

In working with the American Indian family within the health care arena, in addition to employing a holistic approach to health care delivery, a family systems approach is the most effective modality of intervention with American Indian families being confronted with a crisis. A major premise of family systems theory is that the child is an integral member of the larger family unit. All family members interact with one another, thereby influencing the entire family unit. Family systems theory suggests that there are interrelated systems in each family, so the child, the parent, and other family members are all changed by the process of living together. The family functions by providing the child daily care, recreation, socialization, affection, self-definition, educational-vocational training, and economic security, and when some component of this interactive process is not effectively performing, there is a malfunction in the whole system. Family systems theory is well received by the American Indian community, as it recognizes the importance of the entire family and the interrelationship between each component subsystem, as well as the relationship to much larger outside systems, such as the community, the society, and the health care system.

Culture, economics, and personal characteristics shape family characteristics, and this in turn affects the family's response to social challenges brought on by a family crisis, such as chronic illness. Some of the characteristics impacting the family in crisis are family size, coping abilities of the family, and the degree of extended family support. The challenges created by an illness crisis depend upon the severity of the illness, the physical disability involved, and the resultant behavior. Coping ability is related to both the strength of the caretakers as well as the demands of caretaking. Personal traits leading to coping abilities of parents vary greatly. For example, chronic depression in a parent is associated with impaired parenting skills (Paterson, 1992). Knowledge of family functioning is important when the health care professional is developing an intervention plan, and the use of the family systems approach works well when developing such an intervention for an American Indian family. An understanding of family life cycles, which involves the developmental stages, the transitions, and the changes that families undergo as they ebb and flow through life's challenges, also provides a valuable tool for working with American Indian families, because American Indians view life in cycles and can appreciate this concept (DuBray, 1992, 1993). Each cycle has purpose and meaning. Finally, it is important to consider some of the features of challenges faced by American Indian families when confronting a major crisis. These challenges involve changes in interactions within the family system confronted by the crisis. These changes in interactions can lead to re-prioritizing of needs based upon the current needs of the ill family member. This change in functioning can be temporary or long term depending upon the situation. In addition, this adds to the incredible burden already experienced by the American Indian family due to a long history of disenfranchisement and poverty, as well as the historical cultural assault upon the community. Understanding this information would be an important factor in the provision of adequate health care services to the American Indian community.

Today, health care professionals need to be in tune with the impact of stress on families that feel economic and time challenges. The poverty rate among American Indians is extremely high, so these families experience economic stress disproportionately to other groups. Additionally, American Indian families experience intergenerational post-traumatic stress due to the oppressive history of American Indians (Duran & Duran, 1996). Despite the stress, American

Indians care for their elderly, their handicapped, and their children without outside resources. Families that assume such care responsibilities experience even greater stress, by taxing already limited resources and energies, and they need assistance through the provision of services, such as in-home health services, homemaker training, respite care, medical equipment, companionship, and support. Most American Indian families will not request these services from outside agencies, but will simply "make do." Therefore, moving toward a model that sees American Indian families as the primary social service agency allows the health care professional to be in tune with the family's needs and to make sure that the family receives the assistance needed, which will improve health care delivery to American Indian families, thereby resulting in the subsequent reduction of the stresses related to caring for family members. The family systems model offers such an approach to the health care professional.

CULTURALLY SENSITIVE HUMAN SERVICE DELIVERY

Although they frequently appear cooperative, American Indian parents, who have experienced discrimination, usually approach exchanges with Euro-American institutions with a certain reserve (DuBray, 1992; Locke, 1992). American Indian parents are cautious and slow in developing trust, hence they focus on actions rather than words. Health care professionals need to be aware of this and need to factor this into outreach activities in order to provide the families with culturally sensitive information needed to increase their health care access and knowledge base (Clarke, Zales & Sacco, 1982). The health care professionals must make the American Indian family a part of the health care team, and they must share the initial evaluation, the treatment plan, and the course of treatment with the family, thereby demonstrating the desire for collaboration (Anderson & Stewart, 1983; Green, 1982; Sullivan, 1983; Paterson, 1982).

In addition to including the family in all aspects of health care planning, health care professionals need to focus on the strengths of American Indian families instead of the deficits (Clark, Zales & Sacco, 1982; Anderson & Stewart, 1983). Deficits overshadow strengths as chronic illness progresses and functioning of the family deteriorates. Therefore, it is critical to look for strengths within the American Indian family and to validate these strengths by acknowledging them to the family. American Indian families feel the daily stress of a hostile society, and replication of this behavior by the health care staff may jeopardize any progress with the family. One positive method used by Indian Health Services (a division of the United States Department of Health and Human Services, Public Health Services) in the provision of care to American Indian families, both on reservations and in urban areas, is the use of community health representatives. Because they are specially trained members of the Indian community, community health representatives have been successful in bridging the gap in services, and the use of such a worker to conduct outreach could offer a viable alternative for providing health care services, particularly where there are a number of traditional Indians, who remain essentially outside of the standard health care delivery system.

At minimum, outreach services are important in the delivery of health care to the American Indian community, and the outreach workers must absolutely be culturally attuned to the specific tribal community in which they are working. Over and above culturally relevant outreach services, all health care professionals must learn to translate knowledge about a culture into actual intervention (Sue, 1988). They must avoid tendencies to overgeneralize and stereotype. In addition, health care professionals must remain open to guidance from the American Indian family (Montalvo & Guitierrez, 1989). The patient's cultural values, perceptions, and goals should be validated (Tyler et al., 1985). Through the provision of culturally sensitive health care practices, which augments practice with social service delivery, American Indian families that are stressed and disenfranchised can be bolstered, which will ultimately improve the quality of and access to health care (Sparks, 1994). This will result in improved communication and a more positive interaction and partnership between the health care professional and the American Indian family client system.

CONCLUSION

Information has been provided throughout this paper to aid in understanding the cultural values, family and child rearing practices, and communication patterns of American Indian families, and strategies have been offered that if used will improve health care delivery to these American Indian families. With these families, utilizing a family systems model is most effective as it fits their priority of community and family cohesiveness over individualistic goals. In addition, a holistic approach recognizes the interconnectedness of the body, mind, and spirit, an ideology prominently found in the American Indian perspective of life.

Over and above using the family systems model and the holistic approach, health care professionals must recognize the importance of extended family members and be aware of grandparents, aunts, uncles, and others identified as pivotal decision makers within the family. To misunderstand these family ties would limit who is involved in the health care of the Indian client, and it would also pathologize these relationships and create a therapeutic failure (Tyler et al., 1985). Health care professionals, as well as all other human service personnel, must respect cultural pluralism and diversity, build on the strengths of the American Indian family, and provide for individual and social change.

Culture is of great importance to American Indians, and family is at the center of culture. American Indian cultures are also variable, therefore, stereotypes must be avoided. Many challenges lie ahead in the education of health care personnel and in the education of American Indian families in navigating the health care system in order to access necessary services. With the challenge of American Indian health care delivery before us, it is appropriate to keep in mind the words of the great Lakota chief and medicine man, Sitting Bull, as we rise to this challenge: "Let us put our minds together and see what kind of life we can make for our children."

REFERENCES

Allen, P. G. (1991). *Grandmothers of the light: A medicine woman's sourcebook*. Boston, MA: Beacon Press.

Anderson, C. M. & Stewart, S. (1983). *Mastering resistance: A practical guide to family therapy*. New York, NY: Guilford.

Anderson, P. P. & Fenichel, E. S. (1989). *Serving culturally diverse families of infants and toddlers with disabilities*.Washington, D.C.: National Center for Clinical Infant Programs.

Ashford, J. B., LeCroy, C. W., & Lortie, K. L. (1997). *Human behavior in the social environment: A multidimensional perspective*. Pacific Grove, CA: Brooks/Cole Publishing Company.

Benet, S. V. (1943). *Western Star*. New York, NY: Holt, Rinehart & Winston, Inc.

Clark, T., Zales, T., & Stacco, F. C. (1982). *Outreach family therapy*. New York, NY: Jason Aronson.

Crowe, T. A. (Ed.). (1997). *Application of counseling in speech-language pathology and audiology.* Baltimore, MD: Williams & Wilkins.
Debo, A. (1970). *A history of the Indians of the United States.* Norman and London: University of Oklahoma Press.
DuBray, W. (1992). *Human services and American Indians.* St. Paul, MN: West Publishing.
DuBray, W. (1993). *Mental health interventions with people of color.* St. Paul, MN: West Publishing.
Duran, E. & Duran, B. (1996). *Native American-Post Colonial Psychology.* New York, NY: State University of New York.
Garrison, W. T. & McQuiston, S. (1989). *Chronic illness during childhood and adolescence: Psychological aspects.* Newbury Park, CA: Sage Publication.
Green, J. W. (1982). *Cultural awareness in the human services.* Englewood Cliffs, NJ: Prentice-Hall.
Hendren, R. L. & Berline, I. N. (1991). *Psychiatric inpatient care of children and adolescents: A multicultural approach.* New York, NY: John Wiley & Sons, Inc.
LaFromboise, T. (1988). American Indian mental health policy. *American Psychologists, 43,* 388-397.
Lake, M. G. (1991). *Native healer: Initiation into an ancient art.* Wheaton, IL: Quest Books.
Leap, W. L. (1981). American Indian language maintenance. *Annual Review of Anthropology.*
Locke, D. C. (1992). *Increasing multicultural understanding: A comprehensive model.* Newbury Park, CA: Sage Publications.
Lum, D. (1996). *Social work practice and people of color: A process-stage approach.* Pacific Grove, CA: Brooks/Cole Publishing Company.
Montalvo, B. & Guitierrez, M. J. (1989). Nine assumptions for work with ethnic minority families. In G. W. Saba, B. M. Karrer & K. V. Hardy (Eds.). *Minorities and Family Therapy.* Binghamton, NY: The Haworth Press, Inc.
Paterson, R. (1982). *Cohesive family process.* Eugene, OR: Cartalia Publishing.
Sparks, S. (1994). Cycles of rehospitalization. Unpublished masters thesis. California State University, Sacramento, Sacramento, California.
Steer, D. (1996). *Native American Women.* New York, NY: Barnes & Noble Books.
Sue, D. W. & Sue, D. (1990). *Counseling the culturally different: Theory and practice* (2nd ed.). New York, NY: John Wiley.
Sue, S. (1988). Psychotherapeutic services for ethnic minorities: Two decades of research findings. *American Psychologist, 43,* 301-624.
Sullivan, T. (1983). Native children in treatment: Clinical, social and cultural issues. *Journal of Psychoanalytic Anthropology, 1,* 75-94.
Topper, M. D. (1987).The traditional Navajo medicine man: Therapist, counselor and community leaders. *Journal of Psychoanalytic Anthropology, 10,* 217-249.
Trad, P. V. (1987). *Infant and childhood depression.* New York, NY: Wiley.
United States Department of Commerce, Bureau of Census (1990). Washington, D.C.: U. S. Government Printing Office.

Index

Acculturation, 4-5,68-70
American Indian ethnicity, health care and
  acculturation degree and, 68-70, 71-72
  "American Indian" designator and, 70
  conclusions regarding, 82-83
  culture and
    behavioral patterns shaped by, 73-76
    "being" vs. "doing" philosophy and, 75-76
    communication patterns and, 72,73
    community health representatives and, 82
    definition of, 67-68
    family as mediator of, 71-72,83
    group vs. individual and, 74-75
    intrinsic individual worth and, 74
    mistrust of health care professionals and, 73,81
    natural harmony and, 75,76
    passive behavior and, 73
    service delivery sensitivity and, 67,81-82
    time perceptions and, 75,76
  demographics regarding, 70-71
  ethnicity, defined, 68
  extended family and, 70,72, 78-81,83
  family systems intervention and, 82-83
    coping abilities and, 80
    economic stress and, 80
    family characteristics and, 80
    family life cycles and, 80
    intergenerational post-traumatic stress and, 80-81
  natural healing levels and, 77-78
  spirituality and
    Christianity integration and, 78
    cultural identity through, 71
    healing perspective on, 74, 76-77
    holistic approach and, 76,77, 78,79,83
    purposive nature of humanity and, 76
    spiritual leaders and, 77
    summary regarding, 67-68
    Sun Dance ceremony (Lakota) and, 77
  urban lifestyles and, 70-71
American Indian gaming, social impact of
  Grounded Theory study methods and, 26-27
  historic background (Minnesota) on, 24-25
  implications of, 33
  job skills and, 23
  "new buffalo" concept and, 23
  study findings (negative) regarding
    alcohol and drug abuse, 25
    casino gaming, impact of, 28-31
    child care issues, 23,27,30
    depression, 25
    gambling abuse, addiction, 23, 24-25,27,29
    materialism, 23,28,31-32
    poverty, 25,29-30
    tribal culture affected by, 23,27, 28,31-32
    unemployment, 25
  study findings (positive) regarding

employment opportunities,
23-24,27,28-29
negative stereotypes,
breakdown of, 28,30-31
positive collective
consciousness, 27,28
self-worth, 27,28,32
study methods and, 25-27
tribal voices method and, 24
summary regarding, 23-24
American Indian. *See* American
Indian ethnicity, health care
issues and; American Indian
gaming, social impact of;
Human Genome Diversity
Project; Indian Child Welfare
Act; Lakota historical trauma
response
American Indian Studies Center, Los
Angeles, CA, 47
American Type Culture Collection
(ATCC), 54
Assimilated form of acculturation, 69
Association of American Indian and
Alaska Native Social
Workers, 46
ATCC (American Type Culture
Collection), 54

Bicultural form of acculturation, 69

Cavalli-Sforza, Luca, 52,61
Children. *See* Indian Child Welfare
Act
Crania Americana (Morton), 60

Ethnicity. *See* American Indian
ethnicity, health care and
Ezell, Cambria, 59

Gaming. *See* American Indian
gaming, social impact of

Gender differences. *See* Lakota
historical trauma response,
gender differences in
Genes. *See* Human Genome Diversity
Project
Gould, Stephen Jay, 60
Grounded Theory study methods,
26-27

Health care. *See* American Indian
ethnicity, health care issues
and; Human Genome
Diversity Project; Indian
Child Welfare Act; Lakota
historical trauma response
Hettinger, Ned, 55.
HGDP. *See* Human Genome Diversity
Project (HGDP)
Historical trauma response. *See*
Lakota historical trauma
response
Hizfeld Index, 60
Holocaust survivors, 1,2,4,16
Human Genome Diversity Project
(HGDP), 52-53
advantages from
human evolution answers, 51
medical science and technology
advancement, 51
collection methods and, 53-54
conclusions regarding, 62-63
endangered indigenous populations
and, 52
ethical concerns and, 58-59,62-63,
65n. 5
bribery tactics and, 61-62
control over genetic material, 53
denial of information access
and, 52,53,62
fetal and placental tissue
samples and, 59
genetic biological weapons and,
60-61
genetic racial discrimination
and, 60

Index

misuse of genetic information and, 59-60
non-living persons' samples and, 59
inclusion criteria and, 53
patenting and
 cloned genes, defined, 64n. 1
 cultural values and, 58
 genetic imperialism concept and, 58
 human cell line, defined, 63n. 1
 of human genetic material, 55-57
 hybridomas, defined, 64n. 1
 of indigenous peoples' human cell lines, 57-58, 64n. 4
 Limone gene example of, 56
 "Mo Cell" example of, 56,58
 Supreme Court Case regarding, 55-56,64nn. 2,3
policy implications regarding, 58-62,63
profit potential from, 54-55
summary regarding, 51-52

ICWA. *See* Indian Child Welfare Act (ICWA)
Indian Child Welfare Act (ICWA)
 best interest of the child and, 39-40
 child custody proceedings and
 defined, 39
 procedural safeguards and, 38
 context and content of, 38-40
 cultural continuity and, 39-40
 factors leading to
  boarding schools, 36
  foster care placement rates, 36-37,41
  foster home licensing standards, 37
  social service agencies, racism of, 37-38
  unnecessary removals, 37
 funding inadequacy and, 35,36,42
 implementation of
  amendments proposed, 53

 communication deficiencies and, 42-43
 constitutionality issue and, 40
 inconsistencies, ambiguities and, 40
 infrastructure deficiencies and, 40
 in New York State, 43-45
 overcoming roadblocks to, 45-48
 state legislation and, 40
 study of effects of, 40-42
 violations of, 41
"Indian child," defined, 38-39
recommendations regarding
 for administrators and politicians, 48
 for practitioners and human services students, 48-49
summary regarding, 35-36
training needs and, 45-48
Indigenous children. *See* Indian Child Welfare Act

King, Mary-Claire, 53

Lakota Grief Experience Questionnaire (LGEQ), 10-11
Lakota historical trauma response
 features of, 3-4
 Holocaust survivor syndrome and, 1,2,4,16
 impaired or delayed mourning and, 3
 medical and psychosomatic conditions and, 2,4
 mortality rates and, elevation of, 2
 PTSD and, 3
 summary regarding, 1-2
 Wounded Knee Massacre and, 2,3,14
 See also Lakota historical trauma response, gender differences in

Lakota historical trauma response, gender differences in
  acculturation vs. health status and, 4-5
  alcohol abuse and, 6
  boarding schools and, 10-11
  depression and, 6-7
  risk factor of, 8
  tuberculosis and, 7
  childhood sexual abuse and, 5,6
  conclusions regarding, 15-16
  depression and, 5,6,7
  discussion regarding, 14-15
  findings regarding
    boarding school experiences, 10-11,14
    intervention effectiveness, 12-15
    traditional presentation-of-self, 11-12,14-15
  heart and cerebrovascular diseases and, 6,7,9,15
  Lakota Grief Experience Questionnaire and, 10-11
  medical and psychosomatic conditions and, 6-7,15
  psychiatric disorders and, 5-6,15
  PTSD and, 5,6-7,8-9
  risk factors and
    life expectancy, 8
    socioeconomic status, 8
    traditional presentation-of-self, 8-9
  study intervention and methodology and, 9-10
  substance abuse and, 5,6,8
  suicide and, 5-6,8
  Takini (Survivor) Network and, 16
  traditional roles and relationships and, 4-5
  tuberculosis and, 7
  unemployment rate and, 8
LGEQ (Lakota Grief Experience Questionnaire), 10-11

Mismeasure of Man, The (Gould), 60
Morton, Samuel George, 59-60

National Graves Protection and Repatriation Act, 59
New York State Bureau of Indian Services, 44-45

O'Brien, Sharon, 61
Oklahoma Indian Child Welfare Association, 46

Phenotype
  historical trauma response and, 11-12
  as risk factor, 8-9,15-16
Post-traumatic Stress Disorder (PTSD), Lakota historical trauma and, 3,6-7,8-9
Pte Sa Win (White Buffalo Calf Woman, Lakota), 4,14

RAFI (Rural Advancement Foundation International), 54
Rural Advancement Foundation International (RAFI), 54

St. Regis Mohawk Nation, 44-45
Sun Dance ceremony (Lakota), 77

Teton Sioux. *See* Lakota historical trauma response
Traditional form of acculturation, 69
Traditional presentation-of-self
  gender differences in, 8-9
  as historical trauma response risk factor, 8-9
  intervention results and, 12-14

Wilson, Allan, 52
Wounded Knee Massacre, 2,3,14